THE CARBO-CALORIE DIET COOKBOOK

The Carbo-calorie Diet Cookbook

DONALD S. MART

Dolphin Books
Doubleday & Company, Inc., Garden City, New York

Dolphin Edition: 1976

Library of Congress Cataloging in Publication Data
Mart, Donald S
The carbo-calorie diet cookbook.
Based on the author's The carbo-calorie diet published
in 1973.
Includes index.
1. Low-calorie diet. 2. Low-carbohydrate diet.
I. Title.
RM222.2.M3642   641.5′635
ISBN 0-385-09908-8
Library of Congress Catalog Card Number 75–36617

Love to my wife, Beverly, for her devoted help in the compilation of this book, and my special thanks to all of the advocates and readers of *The Carbo-calorie Diet*, the book that made this book possible.

Contents

Recipes for items followed by asterisk may be located by consulting the Index.

Foreword

(taken from *The Carbo-calorie Diet*)

This book should become the standard for dieters throughout the world.

As a practitioner of medicine for many years, I have found that a steadily increasing number of overweight patients have been asking physicians to help them lose weight.

Diets have been prescribed, but in many instances sustained and adequate weight reduction is not accomplished and the diet is abandoned.

It should seem simple, yet why is it that some people cannot lose weight, no matter how little they eat?

I have always believed in a "natural" approach to dieting, whereby the amount of food and the types of food ingested are restricted to the degree that weight will be lost in an orderly and healthful manner.

For many years the calorie was the total judgment of how much a food or beverage could influence the weight of a person and, there being no other guide, was used exclusively. Unfortunately, the calorie diet is quite stringent and, because of the unsatisfying nature of the diet, difficult for many to maintain over any extended period of time.

Not too long ago a new form of diet measurement made itself known—grams of carbohydrate. This diet is almost a direct antithesis of the calorie diet. You can eat many of the "forbidden fruits," and even imbibe of alcoholic beverages without too much fear of adding on weight (or so it is stated). But, how can one diet say that you cannot have this or that, while the other one says you can? How can one diet say that certain foods or alcoholic beverages have absolutely no weight-adding factors, while the other one, to state it quaintly, is loaded with extra poundage? These discrepancies between the two diets have not only split the dieters into two camps, but also many physicians on the merits of each.

Recently, though, I received word of a new unit of diet

measurement and decided to investigate it. I was astounded by the innovativeness and logic of this new concept and wondered why no one else had conceived of the premise. Mr. Donald S. Mart, the author of this book, has developed a formula to *combine* calories and carbohydrates into *one, single* unit of diet measurement to compensate and adjust for the differences between the two diets, yet retain much of their individual and intrinsic values. Simply stated, a person will *automatically* be able to adhere generally, with little or no effort, to both a calorie diet and a carbohydrate diet *simultaneously* on an average over a reasonable period of dieting by utilizing balanced daily diet menus made up from the tables in this book. This new diet is a planned and reasoned program for the systematic loss of weight that should work in almost every case of obesity because of the recognition of the calorie and the carbohydrate as equally important diet factors.

I would like to reiterate that the "carbo-calorie," as Mr. Mart has coined the name for this new unit of diet measurement, should replace the calorie and the carbohydrate and become the new standard for all dieters.

Robert J. Heller, M.D.

Introduction

I

In May of 1973 *The Carbo-calorie Diet* (a Dolphin book) was published. Its ever-increasing popularity has made the writing of this book almost mandatory. People everywhere have requested that a cookbook based on the carbo-calorie diet be prepared so that the diet itself can be more fully utilized.

For those of you who do not have *The Carbo-calorie Diet* with its listings of many thousands of foods and beverages by carbo-calorie count, following is a brief explanation of what the carbo-calorie is and how it can help you lose those ugly pounds.

The basic problem of whether to follow a calorie diet or a carbohydrate diet, and the effectiveness of each, is resolved by the carbo-calorie—a mathematical combining of the calorie count and the carbohydrate gram count of foods and beverages, thereby eliminating the confusion of which diet to use and giving you the benefits of both.

The one major rule to follow when using the carbo-calorie diet is:

EAT 100 CARBO-CALORIES A DAY, OR LESS.

It's as simple as that. One hundred carbo-calories a day, or less, is your diet. It is a realistic diet that takes into account the two most important diet factors. You will find that the diet isn't as happy as an all-carbohydrate diet, but on the other hand, it is nowhere near as stern as a pure calorie diet. This diet regulates your intake of carbohydrates and calories simultaneously, although it is possible on a given day to exceed the limitations of one or the other (but never both). Your daily carbo-calorie diet menus exercised over a reasonable diet span should, to a fair degree, average out any such anomalies. When you've had your carbo-calories for the day you will know that you haven't been a saint with your calorie count but killed yourself with a ton of carbohydrate grams—and vice versa.

The first thing you have to understand is that a carbo-calorie doesn't exist—not in a real sense. The calorie is a unit of heat measurement (to be exact, the amount of heat needed to raise the temperature of one kilogram of water one degree centigrade at sea level) and when used in a diet refers to the energy produced by food when oxidized in the body. A gram of carbohydrate refers to something actually tangible; that is, a gram of any of certain organic compounds composed of carbon, hydrogen, and oxygen, including the sugars, starches, and celluloses.

When you combine a calorie with a gram of carbohydrate it can be done only on a mathematical basis, never on a physical or actual basis. Therefore, as a unit of diet measurement, carbo-calories exist—as a real thing, they do not. With that in mind, here is how the carbo-calorie formula was developed:

The first step was to determine the average calorie diet and the average carbohydrate diet. Many texts and references were studied and a grand total average was made of the diets stated in them. The results showed that a 1,200 calorie diet and a 60-gram carbohydrate diet were about middle-of-the-road between out-and-out starvation diets and pure medical-maintenance diets. These two figures then became the basis for the carbo-calorie formula:

$$\frac{20A+B}{24}=X$$

A is the carbohydrate count, B is the calorie count, and X is the carbo-calorie count.

By applying the above formula, here is how the basic diet of 100 carbo-calories per day was arrived at:

$$\frac{20\times60 \text{ (grams of carbohydrate)}+1200 \text{ (calories)}}{24}=$$
$$100 \text{ CARBO-CALORIES}$$

As a real example, let us use one plain, four-inch pancake, a favorite breakfast food. It contains 9.2 grams of carbohydrate and 64 calories. Applying the foregoing formula leads to this result:

$$\frac{20 \times 9.2 \ (\text{grams of carbohydrate}) + 64 \ (\text{calories})}{24} =$$

10.3 CARBO-CALORIES

This brings out how misleading a calorie diet or a carbohydrate diet can be when used individually. Our pancake has only 64 calories or, in other words, is equivalent to a little over $\frac{1}{20}$ of your day's diet if using a 1,200 calorie diet—so you go blithely along stuffing yourself with those great pancakes, figuring you have plenty of leeway. But, take a look at the carbohydrate side! One pancake is almost $\frac{1}{6}$ of your day's diet, using a 60-gram carbohydrate diet. Pretty shocking, and very often the reason why people have difficulty losing weight when dieting. On the other hand, there are many reverse examples where the carbohydrate count is low but the calories very high. For instance, look at a cooked four-ounce portion of corned beef (average lean and fat) that we have with cabbage or stick in a sandwich; it has absolutely no carbohydrate grams, but does have 422 calories—over $\frac{1}{3}$ of your daily 1,200 calorie diet. Can you picture the imaginary situation of someone on a carbohydrate diet, eating only corned beef all day? As far as that person is concerned, he is on the best diet in the world—no carbohydrates at all—and should be shedding pounds by the bucketful. But, after eating just 12 ounces of corned beef, he is already over the standard 1,200 calorie diet.

The carbo-calorie diet is designed so that one may eat a variety of all types of foods, including carbohydrates, which are severely restricted on high-protein and/or high-fat (low-carbohydrate) diets.

The major problem with low-carbohydrate diets is that when one does eat a food relatively high in carbohydrates, weight gain will result far out of proportion to the caloric values of the food ingested. This is due to a complex interaction of metabolic events leading to salt and water retention, delayed weight loss, and, at times, weight gain. This is not a true fat deposition, but represents excessive weight gain from body water. Thus, a small amount of carbohydrates on a low-carbohydrate diet may lead to weight gain, rather than weight loss, and abandonment of the weight-reduction program.

The carbo-calorie diet, however, does not have to contend with this disadvantage of the low-carbohydrate diet. On the carbo-calorie diet, one may eat carbohydrates and not count calories, and still lose weight as long as one stays within the daily quota of 100 carbo-calories.

While I was developing the carbo-calorie formula, I discovered another important point during the researching of the many texts and documents. Most nutritionists felt that an intake of less than 30 grams of carbohydrate or 800 calories a day could possibly be detrimental to one's health, although under medical supervision there are diets applied that are less than that. For the sake of this general diet, we will use the 30-gram carbohydrate and 800 calorie diets as our minimum. Applying our carbo-calorie formula leads to this result:

$$\frac{20 \times 30 \text{ (grams of carbohydrate)} + 800 \text{ (calories)}}{24} =$$

58.3 CARBO-CALORIES

Therefore, eat at least 58 carbo-calories a day, but don't eat over 100. If you want to lose weight more quickly, instead of planning your menus for a full 100 carbo-calories each day, plan them for, say, 75 carbo-calories a day. This will create an accelerated weight loss, yet still give you the nutritional values your body requires. Remember, you've got to stay healthy and happy when dieting.

II

Now that you have an understanding of what the carbo-calorie diet is, let us put it to practical use. First of all, this book is not intended to show you how to broil a steak, or boil an egg, or open up a can of soup. We assume that you already know how to do that. Instead, you will find recipes that are not run-of-the-mill, recipes that will whet your appetite, recipes that you thought you could never have on a diet.

Preparing a recipe is simply the proper blending of varying amounts of different edible ingredients to make an end product. Because of these varying quantities of different ingredients, very often the calorie, or carbohydrate, or carbo-calorie count gets lost in the shuffle—it is too hard to calculate. To overcome that, the recipes on the following pages show the carbo-calorie count both by total recipe and by individual serving so that you can cook many delicious dishes and also keep track of those all-important carbo-calories.

Except for the substitution of artificial sweetener for sugar and the recommendation that dietetic pack (usually water) canned vegetables or fruits be used, no special dietetic ingredients are used in these recipes. Everything in them can be obtained at your local grocery store. The reason for this is that the carbo-calorie diet is a natural diet, one that allows you to eat every kind of food, whether it contains carbohydrate, protein, or fat—as long as you limit your eating to 100 carbo-calories a day or less.

III

When making up your carbo-calorie menus for the day, try to keep your selection of foods well balanced to maintain a healthy diet. If you have an urge to have a variety of tastes, there is nothing against halving, or even quartering, the recommended individual servings so that you can expand the content of your menus. The following sample menus contain many of the recipes in this book (they are marked with an asterisk *) and show you how great eating can be while losing weight.

Sample Menus

BEAUTIFUL BREAKFASTS

		Carbo-calories
1 serving Cheese Omelet*		12
3 strips bacon		6
1 slice buttered white toast		15
1 cup black coffee (no sugar)		½
	Total	33½

½ serving Ambrosia*		8¾
½ cup corn flakes		9
½ cup milk (for cereal)		8
1 cup black coffee (no sugar)		½
	Total	26¼

1 glass tomato juice (4 ounces)		6
1 piece French Toast*		15
1 pat butter		2
1 teaspoon powdered sugar for French Toast		8
1 serving Creamy Omelet*		9
1 serving ham (4 ounces)		11
1 cup black coffee (no sugar)		½
	Total	51½

½ cup strawberries		7
½ serving Spanish Omelet*		12½
1 serving Veal Kidneys*		11
1 cup black coffee (no sugar)		½
	Total	31

	Carbo-calories
1 serving Scrambled Eggs* (3 eggs)	17
2 pork sausages	11
1 slice buttered wheat toast	14
1 cup black coffee (no sugar)	½
Total	42½

LUSCIOUS LUNCHES

		Carbo-calories
1 serving Chopped Steak (Hamburger)*		14
½ serving Tossed Salad* with Slim Salad Dressing*		10
1 low-calorie soft drink		1
	Total	25
1 Midwest Sandwich*		28
1 dill pickle		3
1 low-calorie soft drink		1
	Total	32
1 Stuffed Tomato with Crab Meat*		10½
1 glass V-8 juice (4 ounces)		5
	Total	15½
1 Hot Ham Sandwich*		32½
1 cup plain tea		½
	Total	33
1 serving Welsh Rarebit*		13
1 serving Spinach Salad* with Bacon Salad Dressing*		14
1 low-calorie soft drink		1
	Total	28
½ serving Creamed Lobster Patties*		14¾
¼ cantaloupe		7
1 cup plain tea		½
	Total	22¼

DELECTABLE DINNERS

		Carbo-calories
1 martini		7
1 Appetizer of Canned Artichoke*		8
1 cup consommé		2
1 glass dry red wine (4 ounces)		5
1 serving Fillet of Beef*		26
1 serving Sauced Brussels Sprouts*		5½
1 cup black coffee (no sugar)		½
	Total	54
½ serving Oyster Stew*		10
1 serving Creamed Crab Meat*		22
1 serving cooked green beans		3
1 glass dry white wine (4 ounces)		5
1 Cup Custard*		9½
	Total	49½
1 serving Vegetable Soup with Meat*		9
1 serving Chicken Fricassee*		27½
1 serving Potatoes on the Half Shell*		13¾
3 carrot sticks		1
1 stalk celery		2
1 cup black coffee (no sugar)		½
	Total	53¾

		Carbo-calories
1 whiskey highball with soda or water		4
½ serving Avocado Salad*		13½
2 broiled scampi in garlic butter		6
1 serving Hungarian Goulash*		23
1 glass champagne (4 ounces)		6
1 cup black coffee (no sugar)		½
	Total	53

1 serving Cheese Soufflé*		19
1 lamb chop (4 ounces)		9
½ cup cauliflower		3
½ cup spinach		3
1 serving Blanc Mange*		12
1 cup black coffee (no sugar)		½
	Total	46½

Recipes

Turn the page to find an exciting world of wonderful recipes—recipes of your favorite dishes, and dishes you've never tried before. With them, and using a little discretion, you will find it quite easy to make up your own interesting menus while staying within 100 carbo-calories a day.

To quote from *The Carbo-calorie Diet*:

"Eat hearty, be merry, and lose inches!"

BREAKFAST DISHES

ASPARAGUS OMELET

Creamy Omelet*
1 cup White Sauce*
1 can cut asparagus

Make Creamy Omelet. Make White Sauce. Add asparagus, drained and rinsed, to the White Sauce, spread some of the mixture over half of the baked omelet, fold over the other half, turn on platter, and pour over the rest of the sauce.

NUMBER OF SERVINGS: 2
TOTAL CARBO-CALORIES: 51
CARBO-CALORIES PER SERVING: 25½

CHEESE OMELET

1 egg
1 tablespoon cream
4 tablespoons grated Parmesan cheese
Salt to taste
¾ teaspoon butter

Beat egg well. Add cream, stir in the cheese and add salt. Place in a dish greased with butter and bake until firm in a moderate oven, about 350° F.

NUMBER OF SERVINGS: 1
TOTAL CARBO-CALORIES: 12
CARBO-CALORIES PER SERVING: 12

CREAMY OMELET

4 eggs
4 tablespoons milk
½ teaspoon salt
⅛ teaspoon pepper
1 teaspoon butter

Beat eggs slightly, enough to blend the yolks and whites. Add milk and seasoning. Put butter in hot skillet; when melted, turn in the mixture. As it cooks, draw the edges toward the center with a knife until the whole is set. If desired, brown underneath by increasing heat. Fold and turn on hot platter.

NUMBER OF SERVINGS: 2
TOTAL CARBO-CALORIES: 18
CARBO-CALORIES PER SERVING: 9

SPANISH OMELET

2 tablespoons butter
1 tablespoon chopped onion
6 olives, chopped
½ green pepper, chopped fine
1¾ cups canned tomatoes
1 large mushroom, sliced
1 tablespoon capers
¼ teaspoon salt
Few grains cayenne
Creamy Omelet*

Heat the butter in a skillet, add the onion, olives, and green pepper, and cook a few minutes, then add the tomatoes and cook until moisture has nearly evaporated. Add mushroom, capers, salt, and cayenne. Make a Creamy Omelet. Before folding the omelet, place spoonful of sauce on center, then fold and pour the rest of the sauce over and around.

NUMBER OF SERVINGS: 2
TOTAL CARBO-CALORIES: 50
CARBO-CALORIES PER SERVING: 25

CREOLE EGGS

1 *tablespoon chopped onion*
1 *tablespoon chopped green pepper*
1 *tablespoon butter*
1 *small can mushrooms*
1 *tablespoon capers*
1 *cup tomatoes, strained*
6 *eggs*
6 *pieces toast*

Let onion and pepper simmer a few minutes in the butter, add the mushrooms, capers, and tomato liquid, heat through. Beat the whole eggs well and cook with the other ingredients, stirring constantly until the eggs are well scrambled. Serve on toast.

NUMBER OF SERVINGS: 6
TOTAL CARBO-CALORIES: 108
CARBO-CALORIES PER SERVING: 18

EGGS À LA BENEDICT

2 *English muffins*
4 *slices boiled ham*
4 *poached eggs*
*Hollandaise Sauce**
1 *black olive, sliced*

Split and toast English muffins. Fry ham and cut in rounds and place on muffins. Slip poached egg on ham. Cover with Hollandaise Sauce. Garnish with olive.

NUMBER OF SERVINGS: 4
TOTAL CARBO-CALORIES: 144
CARBO-CALORIES PER SERVING: 36

EGGS À LA TARCAT

6 hard-cooked eggs
¼ pound ham, chopped
¼ onion, chopped
¼ teaspoon prepared mustard
1 teaspoon salt
A little red pepper
A few leaves lettuce
1 tablespoon mayonnaise

Cut the eggs in half, lengthwise. Remove the yolk. Rub the yolks smooth with the rest of the ingredients and refill the whites of eggs with this ham mixture. Serve cold on lettuce leaves with a little mayonnaise on each egg (optional).

NUMBER OF SERVINGS: 6
TOTAL CARBO-CALORIES: 42
CARBO-CALORIES PER SERVING: 7

EGGS AND SAUSAGE

1 pound link sausage
2 tablespoons fat
3 eggs

Take cold, boiled sausage, skin and slice in ½-inch pieces. Place in frying pan with hot fat; brown on both sides a few minutes, and just before serving add the eggs, beaten slightly; mix and cook until the eggs are set, and serve immediately.

NUMBER OF SERVINGS: 3
TOTAL CARBO-CALORIES: 105
CARBO-CALORIES PER SERVING: 35

EGG TIMBALES

5 eggs
1 cup milk
Speck white pepper
1 teaspoon chopped parsley
1 cup White Sauce*
Butter

Beat the whole eggs till lemon colored, then add rest of the ingredients. Butter timbale forms, fill with mixture, place forms in a pan half filled with water, and bake 15 minutes in moderate oven, 350° F. Serve with White Sauce.

NUMBER OF SERVINGS: 6
TOTAL CARBO-CALORIES: 66
CARBO-CALORIES PER SERVING: 11

POACHED EGGS AND CHEESE

Butter
6 eggs
½ teaspoon salt
¼ teaspoon paprika
6 teaspoons butter
6 tablespoons grated American cheese
Parsley

Butter 6 ramekins and drop a whole egg in each, add salt and paprika, 1 teaspoon butter each, and cover with 1 tablespoon of the cheese. Place ramekins in a pan of hot water (½ inch deep), and bake until the eggs are set. Place under flame and brown quickly. Garnish with parsley.

NUMBER OF SERVINGS: 6
TOTAL CARBO-CALORIES: 33
CARBO-CALORIES PER SERVING: 5½

SCRAMBLED EGGS

3 eggs
⅓ cup milk
½ teaspoon salt
Pinch pepper
1 teaspoon butter

Beat the eggs slightly, add the milk and seasoning. Cook in a hot, buttered frying pan, over slow fire, stirring constantly until thick, or let cook until white is partially set, then stir.

NUMBER OF SERVINGS: 1
TOTAL CARBO-CALORIES: 17
CARBO-CALORIES PER SERVING: 17

SCRAMBLED EGGS AND CORN

1 tablespoon butter
1 medium can corn, drained
1 teaspoon salt
⅛ teaspoon pepper
4 whole eggs, beaten

Melt butter in skillet, add corn, season to taste, and when well heated, add the beaten eggs, stir and scrape carefully from bottom of pan, and cook gently until eggs are set. Serve at once.

NUMBER OF SERVINGS: 2
TOTAL CARBO-CALORIES: 56
CARBO-CALORIES PER SERVING: 28

VENETIAN EGGS

1 tablespoon butter
1 tablespoon chopped onion
½ medium can tomatoes
Small bay leaf
1 teaspoon salt
Artificial sweetener equivalent to 1 teaspoon sugar
Speck paprika
2 eggs
2 pieces toast

Melt butter, add chopped onion, and cook together for a few minutes; add tomatoes, bay leaf, salt, sweetener, paprika. When hot, pour in the whole eggs. When cooked a bit, break them with a fork. Serve on toast.

NUMBER OF SERVINGS: 2
TOTAL CARBO-CALORIES: 36
CARBO-CALORIES PER SERVING: 18

FRENCH TOAST

1 egg
Pinch salt
1 tablespoon cream
4 slices white bread
1½ teaspoons butter

Beat egg well with salt and cream. Dip slice of bread sparingly into this mixture. Fry a light brown on both sides in butter.

NUMBER OF SERVINGS: 4
TOTAL CARBO-CALORIES: 60
CARBO-CALORIES PER SERVING: 15

PANCAKES

2 eggs, separated
½ teaspoon salt
¼ cup flour
1 cup milk
2 tablespoons butter

Stir yolks with the salt and flour until smooth. Add milk gradually, stirring, then fold in the beaten whites. Heat pan, add butter, and when hot, pour in batter to make four pancakes. Let cook slowly and evenly on one side, turn and brown on the other side, or finish baking in oven.

NUMBER OF SERVINGS:	4
TOTAL CARBO-CALORIES:	40
CARBO-CALORIES PER SERVING:	10

FRENCH PANCAKES

1 cup flour
½ teaspoon salt
1½ cups milk
3 eggs, well beaten
1 tablespoon oil or melted butter
Jelly
Powdered sugar

Sift flour and salt, add milk and eggs, beat all together very well. Have skillet hot and for each pancake add 1 teaspoon fat, spread over pan, pour in a little batter, tilt pan back and forth, so batter will spread all over bottom; when brown, turn and brown on other side. Spread each pancake with jelly and roll up and dust with powdered sugar. Serve hot.

NUMBER OF SERVINGS:	8
TOTAL CARBO-CALORIES:	140
CARBO-CALORIES PER SERVING:	17½

GERMAN PANCAKE

3 eggs
½ teaspoon salt
½ cup flour
½ cup milk
2 tablespoons butter
Powdered sugar
Lemon juice

Beat eggs until very light, add salt and flour, and then the milk, beating all the time. Spread bottom and sides of a 10-inch cold frying pan with the butter. Pour in the egg batter, have oven very hot, 450° F., and bake 20 to 25 minutes, gradually reducing the heat. It should puff up at the sides and be crisp and brown. Place on hot platter and serve with powdered sugar and lemon juice. For larger frying pan, double recipe.

NUMBER OF SERVINGS: 2
TOTAL CARBO-CALORIES: 71
CARBO-CALORIES PER SERVING: 35½

WAFFLES

2 cups flour
2 teaspoons baking powder
Artificial sweetener equivalent to 2 tablespoons sugar
½ teaspoon salt
2 eggs, separated
2 cups milk
5 tablespoons melted butter

Sift flour, add baking powder, sweetener, and salt. Sift again. Beat egg whites until stiff but not dry. Set aside. Beat egg yolks, add milk, and mix with dry ingredients with rotary beater only enough to blend them; add melted butter. Fold in the beaten egg whites last. Overbeating will toughen waffles. Cook in waffle iron.

NUMBER OF SERVINGS: 6
TOTAL CARBO-CALORIES: 240
CARBO-CALORIES PER SERVING: 40

APPETIZERS

APPETIZER OF CANNED ARTICHOKE

6 slices artichoke heart
1 can caviar (4 ounces)
1 teaspoon chopped onion
12 stuffed olives, sliced
3 hard-cooked eggs
Mayonnaise

Cover each piece of artichoke with caviar, chopped onion, and stuffed olives, also chopped white of egg and the yolk put through a ricer, and cover with a thin mayonnaise.

NUMBER OF SERVINGS:	6
TOTAL CARBO-CALORIES:	48
CARBO-CALORIES PER SERVING:	8

ASPARAGUS AND DRIED BEEF STICKS

Drain a can of asparagus tips. Trim slices of dried beef or cooked ham the length of asparagus tip. Spread slices with mayonnaise. Place one stalk on each slice. Roll up tightly, fasten roll with toothpicks.

NUMBER OF SERVINGS:	18
TOTAL CARBO-CALORIES:	36
CARBO-CALORIES PER SERVING:	2

CRAB MEAT-STUFFED CELERY STALKS

Flake a 6-ounce can of crab meat. Add 1 tablespoon lemon juice and 3 tablespoons mayonnaise. Fill into grooves of ten celery stalks.

NUMBER OF SERVINGS:	10
TOTAL CARBO-CALORIES:	45
CARBO-CALORIES PER SERVING:	4½

EGG AND CAVIAR ON CELERY ROOT

4 hard-cooked eggs
1 tablespoon caviar
Salt and paprika to taste
4 ounces boiled celery root

While still hot put eggs through ricer. Mix with caviar, salt, and paprika, press in small buttered mold or in a straight-sided glass, set aside for several hours at room temperature to harden. Cut into eight slices. Serve each on slice of boiled celery root.

NUMBER OF SERVINGS:	8
TOTAL CARBO-CALORIES:	40
CARBO-CALORIES PER SERVING:	5

GOOSE LIVER APPETIZER

1 round slice bread
1 pat butter
1 slice fresh tomato
Salt and pepper to taste
1 slice fried goose liver (1 ounce)
1 hard-cooked egg

Toast bread, 1 slice for each person; butter slightly. Place a thick slice of tomato on top of this; season with salt and pepper. On top of this place fried goose liver. Decorate top with yolk and white of egg, chopped separately.

NUMBER OF SERVINGS: 1
TOTAL CARBO-CALORIES: 18
CARBO-CALORIES PER SERVING: 18

MOLDED SARDINE APPETIZER

2 cans boneless, skinless large sardines (8 ounces each)
½ pound butter
Lemon juice and paprika
Top of pineapple
½ pint pimiento olives

Mash sardines with fork, add creamed butter. Mix and season. Set in refrigerator until firm. Mold in shape of pineapple and stick pineapple top into top. Cover sides with olives, sliced crosswise. Let stand in refrigerator about 6 hours.

NUMBER OF SERVINGS: 12
TOTAL CARBO-CALORIES: 198
CARBO-CALORIES PER SERVING: 16½

SARDINE AND ANCHOVY CANAPÉS

1½ tablespoons butter
1 tablespoon anchovy paste
1 tablespoon flour
½ cup white wine
1 can skinless, boneless sardines (8 ounces)
4 slices toast, buttered

Melt butter. Add anchovy paste, mixing to smooth paste. Add flour, stirring constantly, and cook until mixture bubbles. Add wine gradually, then sardines, heating slowly and taking care not to break sardines. Place sardines on toast, pour sauce over. Serve very hot.

NUMBER OF SERVINGS: 4
TOTAL CARBO-CALORIES: 100
CARBO-CALORIES PER SERVING: 25

TOMATO, CHEESE, AND ANCHOVY CANAPÉS

Spread round of toasted bread with butter, then anchovy paste. Place thin slice tomato on top, sprinkle with grated American cheese; place under broiler until cheese is melted and serve hot; garnish with sprigs of parsley.

NUMBER OF SERVINGS:	1
TOTAL CARBO-CALORIES:	18
CARBO-CALORIES PER SERVING:	18

SOUPS

BLACK BEAN SOUP

1 *pint black beans*
2 *tablespoons chopped onion*
3 *tablespoons butter*
2 *stalks celery or celery root, chopped*
2 *teaspoons salt*
⅛ *teaspoon pepper*
2 *tablespoons flour*
1 *lemon*
2 *hard-cooked eggs*

Soak beans overnight; drain and add cold water and rinse thoroughly. Fry the onion in 2 tablespoons butter, put it with the beans, add the celery and 2 quarts water. Cook slowly until the beans are soft, 3 or 4 hours, add more water as it boils away; rub through a strainer, add the seasoning and heat; heat the remaining 1 tablespoon butter in a saucepan, add the flour, then ⅔ cup and then the rest of the hot soup gradually; cut lemon and eggs in thin slices and serve in the soup.

Number of Servings: 8
Total Carbo-calories: 192
Carbo-calories per Serving: 24

CHEESE SOUP

⅓ cup finely chopped onion
4 tablespoons butter
4 tablespoons flour
1½ tablespoons cornstarch
4 cups chicken stock
4 cups milk
1 cup cooked chopped carrots
1 cup cooked chopped celery
⅛ teaspoon paprika
½-pound package American Cheddar cheese, cut fine
Chopped parsley

Sauté onion in butter until tender and glassy. Add flour and cornstarch, blending well. Add stock and milk gradually, stirring constantly. When boiling, add carrots, celery, paprika, and cheese. Cook over low heat until cheese is melted. Add salt, if necessary. Serve hot with finely chopped parsley.

NUMBER OF SERVINGS: 10
TOTAL CARBO-CALORIES: 165
CARBO-CALORIES PER SERVING: 16½

CLAM CHOWDER

1 quart clams
2-inch-square fat salt pork
1 medium onion, sliced
4 cups diced potatoes cut in cubes ¾ inch square
4 cups milk
4 teaspoons butter
⅛ teaspoon pepper
1 teaspoon salt
8 soda crackers, crushed

Pick over and drain the clams to remove the pieces of shells. Reserve liquor. Cut the pork into fine pieces; add the onion, fry 5 minutes, add the cubed potatoes, clam liquor, and water enough to cover. Cook until nearly tender, pour into a sauce-pan, and add the milk, butter, pepper, and salt. When the potatoes are done and the milk is boiling hot, add clams, whole or cut up, and the crackers. Cook 3 minutes longer.

NUMBER OF SERVINGS: 8
TOTAL CARBO-CALORIES: 396
CARBO-CALORIES PER SERVING: 49½

CORN CHOWDER

2 onions, sliced
3 tablespoons butter
2 tablespoons flour
4 potatoes, cut in slices
1 medium can or 2 cups fresh corn, cooked
3 cups scalded milk
Salt and pepper

Fry onions in butter, add flour, stirring often so that onions cannot burn; add 2 cups water and potatoes. Cook until the potatoes are soft; add corn, milk, and seasoning, and cook 5 minutes. Season and serve.

NUMBER OF SERVINGS: 8
TOTAL CARBO-CALORIES: 232
CARBO-CALORIES PER SERVING: 29

CREAM OF POTATO SOUP

3 potatoes
1 quart milk
2 slices onion
3 tablespoons butter
2 tablespoons flour
1½ tablespoons salt
¼ teaspoon celery salt
⅛ tablespoon pepper
Few grains cayenne
1 tablespoon chopped parsley

Cook the potatoes till very soft. Scald the milk and onion in a double boiler. Drain the potatoes; add the milk, having removed the onion. Rub through a strainer and put back into double boiler over the fire. Melt the butter, add the flour and seasoning, stirring all the time. Pour some of the hot potato mixture over the thickening, then return to the boiler and cook 5 minutes. Add chopped parsley and serve hot.

NUMBER OF SERVINGS: 4
TOTAL CARBO-CALORIES: 140
CARBO-CALORIES PER SERVING: 35

MULLIGATAWNY SOUP

2 sour apples, sliced
¼ cup sliced onion
¼ cup diced celery
¼ cup diced carrot
1 cup strained tomatoes
½ green pepper, chopped fine
3 pounds raw chicken
¼ cup butter or drippings
1 tablespoon flour
1 teaspoon curry powder
2 cloves
⅛ teaspoon mace
1 teaspoon chopped parsley
Salt and pepper

Cook apples, vegetables, and chicken in the fat until browned; add flour, curry powder, cloves, and the rest of the ingredients plus 4 quarts cold water, and cook slowly until chicken is tender. Remove chicken and cut the meat in small pieces. Strain soup and rub apples and vegetables through a sieve. Add chicken to strained soup. Season and serve hot.

NUMBER OF SERVINGS: 16
TOTAL CARBO-CALORIES: 252
CARBO-CALORIES PER SERVING: 15¾

OXTAIL SOUP

2 oxtails, split
2 tablespoons cooking fat
3 pounds lean beef
1 tablespoon salt
1 large onion, diced
¼ cup diced celery root
1 tablespoon chopped parsley
3 carrots, diced
2 tablespoons flour

Cut oxtails into small pieces and fry lightly in fat. Put meat and oxtails in kettle, add 5 quarts water and salt. Cover. Let cook slowly about 4 hours. Add vegetables, cook 1 hour longer, reducing stock one half. Strain. Heat fat in skillet, add flour, brown slowly, add 1 cup of soup, blend well, and stir into the remaining stock.

NUMBER OF SERVINGS:	20
TOTAL CARBO-CALORIES:	260
CARBO-CALORIES PER SERVING:	13

OYSTER STEW

1 pint oysters
2 tablespoons butter
2 cups scalded milk
½ teaspoon salt
Paprika

Put oysters in strainer over saucepan; keep the oyster liquor, remove any bits of shell, then add oysters to strained liquor. Add butter, cook slowly until edges of oysters curl (3 to 5 minutes). Add milk and salt. Sprinkle with paprika. Serve at once.

NUMBER OF SERVINGS:	2
TOTAL CARBO-CALORIES:	40
CARBO-CALORIES PER SERVING:	20

VEGETABLE SOUP WITH MEAT

2 pounds shin of beef, with meat
2 teaspoons salt
1 cup tomatoes
½ green pepper, chopped
½ cup shredded cabbage
1 small onion
½ small carrot
1 piece celery root
1 sprig parsley
½ cup peas
Artificial sweetener equivalent to 1 teaspoon sugar

Wipe the meat, cut it into small pieces. Put it with the salt into 2 quarts cold water. Cover and simmer 4 hours; then add tomatoes, the pepper, cabbage, onion, carrot, and celery root, all cut fine, the parsley, peas, and sweetener. Cook 1 hour longer; cool. When ready to use, remove fat. Heat and serve.

NUMBER OF SERVINGS: 8
TOTAL CARBO-CALORIES: 72
CARBO-CALORIES PER SERVING: 9

SALAD DRESSINGS AND SALADS

Salad Dressings

BACON SALAD DRESSING

3 slices bacon
¼ cup vinegar
½ teaspoon salt
Artificial sweetener equivalent to 1 teaspoon sugar

Cut bacon into diced pieces with scissors. Cook slowly until crisp. Stir in vinegar and seasoning. Reheat and pour at once over lettuce, spinach, or any salad greens.

NUMBER OF SERVINGS:	1
TOTAL CARBO-CALORIES:	7
CARBO-CALORIES PER SERVING:	7

CREAM SALAD DRESSING

½ teaspoon cornstarch
½ teaspoon mustard
¼ teaspoon salt
Artificial sweetener equivalent to ½ cup sugar
⅓ cup vinegar
1 egg, slightly beaten
1 cup whipped cream

Mix dry ingredients, add vinegar and egg, beat together and cook slowly over boiling water until it coats the spoon. Before

serving, add cream, whipped stiff. Serve over cabbage or other
leafy vegetables.

Number of Servings: 2
Total Carbo-calories: 49
Carbo-calories per Serving: 24½

FRENCH DRESSING

¼ teaspoon salt
⅛ teaspoon paprika
⅛ teaspoon white pepper
1½ tablespoons vinegar
1½ tablespoons lemon juice
6 tablespoons salad oil

Mix all the ingredients in a bowl and beat until well blended.
Serve cold and use to marinate boiled meats, vegetables, and
salads. If desired, add a few drops of onion juice, or rub bowl
with slice of garlic or onion. Put in bottle and shake well before using.

Number of Servings: 2
Total Carbo-calories: 32
Carbo-calories per Serving: 16

ROQUEFORT CHEESE SALAD DRESSING

¼ pound Roquefort cheese
4 tablespoons cream
½ teaspoon paprika
Salt
3 tablespoons lemon juice

Rub the cheese through a fine sieve, mix gradually with
cream, season, add lemon juice gradually, and mix until well
blended.

Number of Servings: 2
Total Carbo-calories: 31
Carbo-calories per Serving: 15½

SLIM SALAD DRESSING

¼ teaspoon salt
¼ teaspoon mustard
⅛ teaspoon pepper
Artificial sweetener equivalent to 2 tablespoons sugar
1 tablespoon chopped onion
2 tablespoons vinegar
2 tablespoons lemon juice

Mix all ingredients, set aside, and keep very cold; pour over salad just before serving. If vinegar is very strong, add water.

NUMBER OF SERVINGS: 1
TOTAL CARBO-CALORIES: 4¼
CARBO-CALORIES PER SERVING: 4¼

SOUR CREAM SALAD DRESSING

½ cup sour cream
1 tablespoon vinegar
1 tablespoon lemon juice
Artificial sweetener equivalent to ½ teaspoon sugar
⅛ teaspoon salt
A little pepper

Beat cream, add vinegar, lemon juice, then seasoning. Mix well.

NUMBER OF SERVINGS: 1
TOTAL CARBO-CALORIES: 14
CARBO-CALORIES PER SERVING: 14

TASTY SALAD DRESSING

Artificial sweetener equivalent to 1 teaspoon sugar
¼ teaspoon salt
¼ teaspoon paprika
3 tablespoons olive oil
1 tablespoon vinegar or lemon juice
2 tablespoons chili sauce
1 clove garlic, minced

Beat all ingredients until well blended. Bottle and place in refrigerator. Use over lettuce and fresh, leafy vegetables. Shake well before using.

NUMBER OF SERVINGS:	2
TOTAL CARBO-CALORIES:	26
CARBO-CALORIES PER SERVING:	13

THOUSAND ISLAND DRESSING

2 tablespoons finely cut green peppers
2 tablespoons finely cut pimiento
1 teaspoon onion juice
1 hard-cooked egg, chopped
1 teaspoon Worcestershire sauce
1 tablespoon catsup
2 tablespoons chili sauce
Salt and paprika
1 cup mayonnaise
¾ cup whipped cream

Mix the first seven ingredients, add a little salt and paprika, blend thoroughly with the mayonnaise, and fold in the whipped cream. Serve ice cold over any salad.

NUMBER OF SERVINGS:	8
TOTAL CARBO-CALORIES:	132
CARBO-CALORIES PER SERVING:	16

VINAIGRETTE DRESSING

6 tablespoons olive oil
3 tablespoons tarragon vinegar
1 hard-cooked egg, riced
Few grains paprika
1 teaspoon minced chives or ½ teaspoon onion juice
1 teaspoon salt
2 tablespoons chopped parsley
½ red pepper or canned pimiento, chopped

Mix together and beat well.

NUMBER OF SERVINGS:	1
TOTAL CARBO-CALORIES:	14
CARBO-CALORIES PER SERVING:	14

SALADS

AVOCADO RING

1 package lime or lemon gelatin
1 cup mayonnaise
3 tablespoons lemon juice
1 teaspoon salt
1 cup mashed avocado
1 cup whipped cream

Pour 1 cup boiling water over gelatin powder. Let thicken, then add other ingredients. Pour into a 7-cup ring mold. Set aside to harden and chill. Serve on shredded lettuce surrounded with any desired salad dressing.

NUMBER OF SERVINGS:	7
TOTAL CARBO-CALORIES:	175
CARBO-CALORIES PER SERVING:	25

AVOCADO SALAD

1 avocado
2 slices fresh pineapple
Lettuce
1 teaspoon salt
¼ teaspoon paprika
2 tablespoons lemon juice
1 teaspoon lime juice

Peel avocado and cut pulp into small pieces. Cut pineapple into cubes. Have twice as much avocado as pineapple. Arrange on crisp head lettuce leaves. Mix other ingredients and pour over fruit.

NUMBER OF SERVINGS: 2
TOTAL CARBO-CALORIES: 54
CARBO-CALORIES PER SERVING: 27

BEAN SALAD

1 pound wax beans
2 eggs
Artificial sweetener equivalent to 2 tablespoons sugar
¼ cup tarragon or malt vinegar
½ pint sour cream
½ cup hot bean liquid

Wash, string, and slice beans. Cook until tender; save cooking liquid. Beat eggs well with the sweetener, vinegar, and sour cream. Mix well. Then add the hot bean liquid, beating well while adding so it will not curdle. Mix with the beans and place in glass jar in the refrigerator. This will keep for several days.

NUMBER OF SERVINGS: 4
TOTAL CARBO-CALORIES: 68
CARBO-CALORIES PER SERVING: 17

BIRD'S NEST SALAD

½ pound cottage cheese
Salt and pepper
1 tablespoon cream
¼ pound nut meats, chopped
1 teaspoon chopped parsley
1 head lettuce
½ cup mayonnaise

Mix cheese to a smooth paste with salt, pepper, and a little cream, add nut meats and parsley, form into balls the size of a hickory nut. Allow 3 or 4 balls for each plate and place in center of crisp lettuce leaves. Add mayonnaise and serve cold.

NUMBER OF SERVINGS: 4
TOTAL CARBO-CALORIES: 114
CARBO-CALORIES PER SERVING: 28½

CARROT, CABBAGE, AND PINEAPPLE SALAD

1 cup shredded cabbage
⅔ cup grated raw carrot
1 cup diced canned pineapple
Cream Salad Dressing*
¼ cup walnuts or pecans

Mix the first three ingredients with Cream Salad Dressing. Sprinkle broken nuts on top.

NUMBER OF SERVINGS: 2
TOTAL CARBO-CALORIES: 51
CARBO-CALORIES PER SERVING: 25½

CHEESE RING

½ pound cottage cheese
Salt and paprika
1 tablespoon gelatin
2 teaspoons chopped chives or green peppers
1 pint whipped cream
1 cup mayonnaise

Mash the cottage cheese until smooth. Season to taste. Moisten gelatin in a little cold water. Dissolve over hot water. Cool. Combine all ingredients and beat until light. Place in ring mold and chill. Remove from mold, place mayonnaise in center.

NUMBER OF SERVINGS: 8
TOTAL CARBO-CALORIES: 98
CARBO-CALORIES PER SERVING: 12¼

CHICKEN SALAD

1 pint diced, cooked chicken
1 cup diced celery
French Dressing*
1 cup mayonnaise
½ cup whipped cream
Lettuce
6 olives
2 hard-cooked eggs
6 radish roses

Mix chicken with celery. Marinate with French Dressing. Chill for several hours. Drain. Before serving, mix well with mayonnaise, to which whipped cream has been added. Serve on crisp lettuce leaves. Decorate with olives, slices of hard-cooked eggs, and radish roses.

NUMBER OF SERVINGS: 4
TOTAL CARBO-CALORIES: 136
CARBO-CALORIES PER SERVING: 34

COLE SLAW

Remove outer leaves from medium-sized cabbage. Shred cabbage very fine. Mix with French Dressing*.

NUMBER OF SERVINGS: 4
TOTAL CARBO-CALORIES: 20
CARBO-CALORIES PER SERVING: 5

CRAB MEAT SALAD

1 can crab meat (1 pound)
4 hard-cooked eggs
¼ cup almonds
1 pint heavy cream
1 cup mayonnaise
Salt and paprika
Head lettuce
1 green pepper or pimiento

Cut the crab meat into large pieces. Cut the whites of the eggs into cubes. Blanch the almonds and cut into thin, lengthwise strips. Mix these ingredients. Whip the cream very stiff, fold into the mayonnaise, add salt and paprika. Add to crab mixture. Serve on salad plates on crisp lettuce; garnish with strips of green pepper or pimiento and top with riced egg yolk.

NUMBER OF SERVINGS: 6
TOTAL CARBO-CALORIES: 186
CARBO-CALORIES PER SERVING: 31

MIXED OR TOSSED SALAD

½ head lettuce
½ bunch water cress
½ head romaine
2 small green onions
6 small radishes
1 medium cucumber
2 medium tomatoes
1 medium avocado

Have greens very crisp, and cut or pull into pieces. Slice onions, radishes, and cucumber and add to greens. Then add the tomatoes, peeled and cut into quarters, and the sliced avocado. Add choice of dressing, mix thoroughly, and serve in a large bowl.

NUMBER OF SERVINGS: 4
TOTAL CARBO-CALORIES: 64
CARBO-CALORIES PER SERVING: 16

SALMON MOLD

½ tablespoon salt
Artificial sweetener equivalent to 1½ teaspoons sugar
1 teaspoon dry mustard
¾ cup scalded milk
1½ tablespoons melted butter
2 egg yolks, beaten
¼ cup hot vinegar
¾ tablespoon gelatin
2 tablespoons cold water
1 can salmon (1 pound)

Mix dry ingredients well with milk in double boiler, stir and cook 5 minutes. Add the melted butter, the yolks, beaten with 1 tablespoon of cold water, and the hot vinegar. Stir and cook a moment. Then add gelatin, softened in 2 tablespoons of cold water for 2 minutes. Stir until dissolved, add the salmon, and turn into small molds or ring mold to harden.

NUMBER OF SERVINGS: 6
TOTAL CARBO-CALORIES: 66
CARBO-CALORIES PER SERVING: 11

SALMON OR TUNA FISH SALAD

1 large can salmon or tuna fish
2 cups chopped celery
1 medium green pepper, chopped
1 cup mayonnaise
Lettuce
Paprika

Break up tuna or salmon, add celery, green pepper, and mayonnaise, blending well. Have everything ice cold. Arrange on lettuce leaves and sprinkle with paprika.

NUMBER OF SERVINGS: 4
TOTAL CARBO-CALORIES: 120
CARBO-CALORIES PER SERVING: 30

SPINACH SALAD

Pick young, tender leaves off spinach, wash carefully, and mix with French Dressing*, adding, if desired, finely chopped crisp bacon or Bacon Salad Dressing*.

NUMBER OF SERVINGS: 2
TOTAL CARBO-CALORIES: 14
CARBO-CALORIES PER SERVING: 7

STUFFED TOMATO SALAD WITH CUCUMBERS

6 ripe tomatoes
2 medium cucumbers
Salt and pepper
1 cup Sour Cream Salad Dressing*
Finely chopped parsley
Lettuce

Scald the tomatoes so that the skins can be easily removed. Cut a slice from the top of each, and with a small spoon scoop out center. Peel the cucumbers, dice them, season highly, and mix with at least half the dressing. Fill the tomato cups with this, and put another spoonful of the dressing on top. Sprinkle parsley over and serve on a bed of lettuce leaves.

NUMBER OF SERVINGS: 6
TOTAL CARBO-CALORIES: 90
CARBO-CALORIES PER SERVING: 15

STUFFED TOMATO SALAD WITH CRAB MEAT

Stuff 6 ripe tomatoes with equal parts of shredded crab meat and caviar; cover with mayonnaise.

NUMBER OF SERVINGS: 6
TOTAL CARBO-CALORIES: 69
CARBO-CALORIES PER SERVING: 11½

WALDORF SALAD

Lettuce
2 cups cut-up celery
2 cups sliced apples
1 cup mayonnaise
1 cup broken pecan and walnut meats

Clean lettuce and keep crisp. When ready to serve, add the celery; remove core and skin of apples, cut in slices, and dice. Mix the celery and apple with mayonnaise. Fold in the nuts. Serve on lettuce.

NUMBER OF SERVINGS: 6
TOTAL CARBO-CALORIES: 192
CARBO-CALORIES PER SERVING: 32

WATER LILY SALAD

6 hard-cooked eggs
1 head lettuce
¼ cup green olives
1 bunch red radishes
Water cress
1 cup French Dressing*

Remove shells from eggs. Roll while warm to flatten ends. Cut each egg around the middle, in deep points, through the whites, at equal distances from each other and from the top and bottom of egg; each half thus fits into the other half and forms the petals. Remove yolks, rice; place egg white halves on shredded lettuce leaves, on a large platter, far apart. To represent buds, scatter olives and radishes which have been cut from the top in the egg white sections. Surround platter with water cress and serve with French Dressing.

NUMBER OF SERVINGS: 6
TOTAL CARBO-CALORIES: 63
CARBO-CALORIES PER SERVING: 10½

CHEESE DISHES

BAKED CHEESE FONDUE

2 cups soft bread crumbs
1 cup milk
¾ cup grated cheese
4 tablespoons butter
1 teaspoon salt
4 eggs, separated

Heat first 5 ingredients in double boiler until cheese is melted. Remove from fire and cool slightly. Add beaten yolks. Fold in beaten whites. Pour into buttered baking dish. Bake in moderate oven, 350° F., about 30 minutes until firm. Serve from dish in which it was baked.

NUMBER OF SERVINGS:	6
TOTAL CARBO-CALORIES:	204
CARBO-CALORIES PER SERVING:	34

CHEESE SOUFFLÉ

2 tablespoons butter
2 tablespoons flour
2 cups hot milk
½ teaspoon salt
½ cup grated cheese
4 eggs, separated

Rub butter and flour together over the fire. When they bubble, gradually add the milk. Season. Add cheese. When melted, remove from fire. Cool. When lukewarm, add beaten yolks, then fold in beaten whites. Pour into buttered baking dish. Bake at 350° F. for 45 minutes or over hot water for 45 minutes to 1 hour or until a knife inserted comes out clean. Heat may be increased during last 15 minutes. Serve at once.

NUMBER OF SERVINGS:　　　　　　　4
TOTAL CARBO-CALORIES:　　　　　　76
CARBO-CALORIES PER SERVING:　19

CHEESE STICKS

2 tablespoons butter
⅔ cup flour
1 cup fresh bread crumbs
1 cup grated American cheese
¼ teaspoon salt
⅛ teaspoon white pepper
Pinch cayenne
2 tablespoons milk

Cream butter, add flour, crumbs, cheese, and seasonings. Mix thoroughly, then add milk. Roll ¼ inch thick, ¼ inch wide, and 6 inches long. Bake until brown in a moderately hot oven, 325° F.

NUMBER OF SERVINGS:　　　　　　　8
TOTAL CARBO-CALORIES:　　　　　112
CARBO-CALORIES PER SERVING:　14

RINKTUM-DITY

1 medium can tomatoes
1 cup grated cheese
½ small onion, grated
1 green pepper, chopped
1 teaspoon salt
2 tablespoons butter
2 eggs
4 pieces white toast

Mix tomatoes, cheese, onion, pepper, and salt. Melt the butter in double boiler, add the mixture, and when heated, add the eggs, well beaten. Cook until eggs are of creamy consistency, stirring and scraping from bottom of pan. Serve on toast.

NUMBER OF SERVINGS: 4
TOTAL CARBO-CALORIES: 84
CARBO-CALORIES PER SERVING: 21

WELSH RAREBIT

1 tablespoon butter
½ pound Cheddar cheese
⅛ teaspoon salt
⅛ teaspoon mustard
Pinch cayenne
1 egg
¼ cup milk
4 slices white toast

Melt the butter, break the cheese into small pieces, and add the cheese and seasoning to the butter. Beat the egg with the milk and add to cheese when it melts, and cook 1 minute. Serve at once on toast.

NUMBER OF SERVINGS: 4
TOTAL CARBO-CALORIES: 52
CARBO-CALORIES PER SERVING: 13

SAUCES

BARBECUE SAUCE

1 cup diced onion or 1 clove garlic
2 tablespoons fat
1 cup chopped tomato
1 cup diced green pepper
1 cup diced celery
2 tablespoons brown sugar
½ tablespoon dry mustard
2 cups stock from roast or soup, or water with meat cubes
Salt and pepper to taste
1 cup catsup

Fry the onion or garlic slightly in fat, add the rest of ingredients, cook slowly 1 hour. Liquid should be reduced about one half and sauce should be well blended. Dip any meat except fowl in sauce before roasting or broiling, or baste with sauce during roasting.

NUMBER OF SERVINGS: 12
TOTAL CARBO-CALORIES: 162
CARBO-CALORIES PER SERVING: 13½

BÉARNAISE SAUCE

2 green onions
2 tablespoons tarragon vinegar
4 egg yolks
4 tablespoons butter
1 tablespoon soup stock
½ teaspoon salt
⅛ teaspoon paprika
1 teaspoon finely chopped parsley

Chop onion, add vinegar, bring to boiling point, let simmer until reduced one half, strain and cool. Add yolks one at a time and stir. Cook slowly until smooth, stirring constantly; add butter gradually, stir, add soup stock and seasoning. Serve hot with broiled meat or fish.

NUMBER OF SERVINGS: 4
TOTAL CARBO-CALORIES: 32
CARBO-CALORIES PER SERVING: 8

BROWN SAUCE (GRAVY)

2 tablespoons butter or fat
1 small onion, chopped (optional)
2 tablespoons flour
1 cup water, meat, fish, or vegetable stock
½ teaspoon salt
⅛ teaspoon pepper

Brown the butter or fat and, if desired, add a small onion, chopped, and when brown add the flour. Let brown, then add ⅔ cup of the liquid at once and the rest gradually. Season. Cook 5 minutes or until thickened. Serve over hot meat, vegetables, dumplings, etc.

NUMBER OF SERVINGS: 4
TOTAL CARBO-CALORIES: 20
CARBO-CALORIES PER SERVING: 5

COCKTAIL SAUCE FOR SEA FOODS

½ cup tomato catsup
2 teaspoons prepared mustard
2 tablespoons lemon juice
1 tablespoon Worcestershire sauce

Mix ingredients and let stand 15 minutes. Serve ice cold over shrimp, oysters, lobster, or crab meat. Add a few drops of Tabasco sauce and horseradish, if desired.

NUMBER OF SERVINGS: 4
TOTAL CARBO-CALORIES: 40
CARBO-CALORIES PER SERVING: 10

HOLLANDAISE SAUCE

½ cup butter
2 egg yolks
1 tablespoon lemon juice
¼ teaspoon salt
A few grains cayenne

With a wooden spoon, rub the butter to a cream, add the yolks, one at a time. Beat well, add the lemon juice, salt, and pepper. About 5 minutes before serving add ½ cup boiling water, and stir rapidly. Cook over water or in double boiler, stirring constantly until it thickens.

NUMBER OF SERVINGS: 6
TOTAL CARBO-CALORIES: 78
CARBO-CALORIES PER SERVING: 13

ITALIAN TOMATO SAUCE

1 onion, finely chopped
1 clove garlic, finely chopped
1 tablespoon oil
1 quart tomatoes, strained
Salt and pepper to taste

Fry onion and garlic in oil until light brown, add tomatoes and seasoning, let cook 30 minutes or until slightly thickened.

NUMBER OF SERVINGS: 8
TOTAL CARBO-CALORIES: 42
CARBO-CALORIES PER SERVING: 5¼

TARTAR SAUCE

1 tablespoon chopped capers
1 tablespoon tarragon vinegar
1 tablespoon chopped olives
1 tablespoon cucumber pickles
1 cup mayonniase

Add all of the ingredients to mayonnaise. Serve cold with fish or cold meat dishes. Add minced chives or onions if desired.

NUMBER OF SERVINGS: 12
TOTAL CARBO-CALORIES: 84
CARBO-CALORIES PER SERVING: 7

WHITE SAUCE FOR VEGETABLES, MEATS, AND FISH

2 tablespoons butter
2 tablespoons flour
1 cup hot milk or cream
⅛ teaspoon pepper
¼ teaspoon salt

Melt the butter in a saucepan. Remove from fire and mix with flour. Cook until it bubbles, then add ⅔ of the hot milk at once and the rest gradually and boil, stirring constantly, until the mixture thickens. Season and serve hot.

NUMBER OF SERVINGS: 4
TOTAL CARBO-CALORIES: 36
CARBO-CALORIES PER SERVING: 9

FISH AND SEA FOOD

FRIED FISH CAKES

1 cup shredded, cold boiled fish
1 cup cold mashed potatoes
Celery salt
Pepper
1 egg, beaten
2 tablespoons melted butter

Mix fish and potatoes, season with salt and pepper, add beaten egg, shape into small cakes, and cook in skillet with butter until nicely browned on both sides.

NUMBER OF SERVINGS:	2
TOTAL CARBO-CALORIES:	48
CARBO-CALORIES PER SERVING:	24

BAKED BLACK BASS

2 pounds black bass
Salt
¼ cup butter
Pepper
2 tablespoons flour
⅓ cup strained tomatoes or 1 sliced fresh tomato
Drawn butter with lemon
Parsley or cress

Clean and wash fish. Sprinkle with salt inside and out and let stand several hours. Put in a pan across which you have placed strips of cloth with which to lift out when cooked. Rub it over with soft butter and a little pepper. Dredge with flour. Put in a hot oven, 450° F., without water in the pan. Baste with hot water when brown; add tomato. When done, remove carefully and place on a hot platter. Draw out the strings and skewers, wipe off the water or fat that runs from the fish, serve with drawn butter flavored with lemon. Garnish with parsley or cress.

NUMBER OF SERVINGS: 4
TOTAL CARBO-CALORIES: 104
CARBO-CALORIES PER SERVING: 26

BAKED HALIBUT WITH CHEESE

2 pounds halibut steaks
2 tablespoons lemon juice
4 tablespoons butter
4 tablespoons flour
2 cups hot milk
Salt and pepper
¾ cup grated American cheese
3 tablespoons Parmesan cheese

Broil halibut steaks about 15 minutes, break into rather large pieces, and place in a buttered baking dish. Sprinkle with lemon juice; make a white sauce of the next five ingredients, and pour over fish. Add grated American and Parmesan cheese, and bake uncovered in moderate oven, 350° F., for 20 minutes. Serve in the baking dish.

NUMBER OF SERVINGS: 6
TOTAL CARBO-CALORIES: 99
CARBO-CALORIES PER SERVING: 16½

BOILED FISH

3 pounds fish, cut in slices and sprinkled with salt
2 tablespoons vinegar
¼ teaspoon whole pepper
1 tablespoon minced onion
1 tablespoon minced celery
1 tablespoon minced carrot

Clean fish and let stand in salt several hours. Let 1 quart water, vinegar, pepper, and vegetables boil until the water is well flavored. Add the fish, a few slices at a time, and let simmer until the flesh is firm and leaves the bones. Remove bones. Place on platter. Strain and reserve the fish stock, if wanted.

NUMBER OF SERVINGS: 8
TOTAL CARBO-CALORIES: 98
CARBO-CALORIES PER SERVING: 12¼

RED SNAPPER WITH TOMATO SAUCE

3 pounds red snapper
Salt and pepper to taste
2 medium onions, sliced
1 medium carrot, diced
½ cup diced celery
2 tablespoons butter
1 cup strained tomatoes
1 tablespoon flour
1 cup sweet cream
Chopped parsley

Clean and bone fish; salt and pepper and let stand several hours. Place onions, carrot, and celery in kettle with 1 quart cold water. Let boil, then add fish, whole or in slices, and the butter and tomatoes. Let cook slowly until flesh is firm or separates easily from bone. Lay carefully on platter. Strain liquid, let heat, add flour dissolved in the cream, let cook until smooth. Pour over fish and serve hot. Garnish with chopped parsley.

NUMBER OF SERVINGS: 6
TOTAL CARBO-CALORIES: 144
CARBO-CALORIES PER SERVING: 24

CANNED SALMON LOAF OR PUDDING

1 can salmon steak (7 ounces)
1 tablespoon butter
1 cup hot milk
1 cup bread crumbs
Salt and pepper
2 well-beaten eggs
White Sauce*

Reserve liquid from salmon and mash fish fine. Melt butter in milk and add bread crumbs and seasonings. Combine with the fish. Lastly, add the eggs. Put into a buttered deep baking dish or custard cups, and steam 1 hour. Turn out onto platter and pour White Sauce over, using the liquid from the salmon with the milk in making the sauce.

NUMBER OF SERVINGS: 3
TOTAL CARBO-CALORIES: 102
CARBO-CALORIES PER SERVING: 34

SALMON TROUT BOILED

3½ pounds salmon trout
2 egg yolks
½ cup cream
1 tablespoon sherry
Parsley

Boil fish in 2 quarts water until the flesh separates from the bones. Place fish on platter. Strain the fish liquid. Beat yolks well, add cream. Pour the egg mixture, gradually, into the hot fish liquid, stirring constantly, then add the sherry. Pour mixture over the fish, then set in oven with oven door open to keep hot. If left too long in oven or if oven is too hot, it will curdle. Serve garnished with parsley.

NUMBER OF SERVINGS: 7
TOTAL CARBO-CALORIES: 126
CARBO-CALORIES PER SERVING: 18

SALMON WITH HORSERADISH SAUCE

3 pounds fresh salmon
Salt
¼ cup melted butter
1 tablespoon chopped parsley
½ pound horseradish root
1 pint cream, beaten stiff

Clean fish, bone, salt, and let stand several hours. Place in fish kettle with boiling salt water (1 teaspoon salt to 1 quart water), and let boil ½ hour or until well cooked. Lift out carefully, place on hot platter, and pour over the melted butter and sprinkle well with the parsley. Serve in a separate bowl the following sauce, 1 large spoonful with each portion of fish: Peel horseradish root, grate, and mix well with the pint of cream. The fish must be hot and the sauce cold.

NUMBER OF SERVINGS: 8
TOTAL CARBO-CALORIES: 238
CARBO-CALORIES PER SERVING: 29¾

BAKED TROUT

3½ pounds trout
1 tablespoon flour
2 cups canned tomatoes
1 medium onion, cut fine
1 piece celery root
1 tablespoon butter
1 egg yolk
½ cup cream or evaporated milk
½ teaspoon Worcestershire sauce

Salt fish and let stand several hours. Wet the flour with a little cold tomato. Place fish in dripping pan with tomatoes, onion, celery, and butter, and bake ½ hour. Strain the sauce and just before sending to the table, thicken with egg yolk mixed with the cream, and add Worcestershire sauce.

NUMBER OF SERVINGS: 7
TOTAL CARBO-CALORIES: 157½
CARBO-CALORIES PER SERVING: 22½

TUNA À LA KING

1 can tuna (13 ounces)
2 cups White Sauce*
1 teaspoon Worcestershire sauce
½ large green pepper in strips
1 canned pimiento, diced
Salt and pepper to taste

Drain tuna, rinse, and flake. Stir White Sauce until smooth, add Worcestershire sauce, the green pepper, and the pimiento. Mix until smooth, add tuna, salt, and pepper. Cook until thoroughly heated, and serve.

NUMBER OF SERVINGS: 4
TOTAL CARBO-CALORIES: 254
CARBO-CALORIES PER SERVING: 63½

CRAB MEAT IN RAMEKINS OR CASSEROLE

2 tablespoons butter
2 tablespoons flour
1 cup chicken soup
2 egg yolks
1 cup crab meat
½ cup mushrooms
2 tablespoons sherry
Salt and paprika
Buttered bread crumbs

Melt butter, add flour, and when it bubbles add the soup stock and cook until thick and smooth. Beat yolks slightly, add a little of the hot sauce and then gradually the remaining sauce. Add the crab meat and the mushrooms cut in pieces, wine, and seasoning. Heat thoroughly and serve in heated patty shells or baked in ramekins or a casserole, covering top with buttered bread crumbs.

NUMBER OF SERVINGS: 4
TOTAL CARBO-CALORIES: 42
CARBO-CALORIES PER SERVING: 10½

CREAMED CRAB MEAT

2 tablespoons butter
½ cup bread crumbs
1 cup cream
½ teaspoon dry mustard
1 pint crab meat
2 egg yolks, beaten
Salt and cayenne
Tabasco sauce to taste
4 slices white toast

Mix and heat the first four ingredients; then add the next four. Serve on toast.

NUMBER OF SERVINGS: 4
TOTAL CARBO-CALORIES: 88
CARBO-CALORIES PER SERVING: 22

CLAMS À LA ST. LOUIS

1 onion, chopped fine
2 tablespoons butter
1 tablespoon flour
30 clams, chopped
Salt and pepper
½ teaspoon red pepper
½ teaspoon mustard
4 egg yolks
12 fresh mushrooms, sautéed
Parsley and truffles

Fry the onion in the butter, adding flour, stirring well; then add clams. Season with salt, peppers, and mustard. Cook for 30 minutes, remove from fire, add egg yolks slightly beaten with 2 tablespoons cold water. Reheat, garnish with mushrooms, parsley, and truffles.

NUMBER OF SERVINGS: 5
TOTAL CARBO-CALORIES: 110
CARBO-CALORIES PER SERVING: 22

FROG LEGS À LA NEWBURG

Boil 2 pounds frog legs in salt water and drain. Heat 2 tablespoons butter, add ½ cup soup stock, ½ cup Madeira wine, salt, and cayenne pepper to taste. Boil 3 minutes. Add ½ pint cream and 3 egg yolks, slightly beaten. Cook 2 minutes, stirring constantly, and pour over frog legs.

NUMBER OF SERVINGS: 4
TOTAL CARBO-CALORIES: 80
CARBO-CALORIES PER SERVING: 20

CREAMED LOBSTER PATTIES

3 tablespoons butter
½ small onion, sliced
½ tablespoon minced green pepper
Dash cayenne
½ teaspoon salt
1 tablespoon minced parsley
1 tablespoon chopped pimiento
1 cup mushrooms in pieces
2 tablespoons flour
2½ cups milk
2 cups diced boiled lobster
2 egg yolks, beaten

Melt butter, add onion, green pepper, cayenne pepper, salt, parsley, pimiento, and mushrooms; stir and cook 10 minutes. Add flour, mix, and pour in gradually 2 cups of milk. Add lobster and cook 10 minutes. Add remaining milk to beaten yolks, and just before serving pour into the lobster mixture. Let cook through without boiling and serve at once in heated patty shells.

NUMBER OF SERVINGS:	4
TOTAL CARBO-CALORIES:	118
CARBO-CALORIES PER SERVING:	29½

LOBSTER À LA BORDELAISE

1 small onion, chopped fine
1 small piece carrot, chopped fine
1 cup White Sauce*
1½ pounds boiled lobster, cut up
Salt and cayenne
¼ cup sherry

Cook the onion and carrot in the White Sauce, add the rest, the sherry last.

NUMBER OF SERVINGS:	2
TOTAL CARBO-CALORIES:	73
CARBO-CALORIES PER SERVING:	36½

LOBSTER À LA NEWBURG

2 boiled lobsters
2 tablespoons butter
¼ teaspoon each grated onion, red pepper, and salt
2 small truffles (optional)
¼ cup sherry or Madeira
3 egg yolks
1 cup cream

Cut lobster in 1-inch pieces. Place in a saucepan the butter, onion, pepper, salt, and the truffles cut in small pieces, and cook for 5 minutes; add the wine and cook 3 minutes. Have the yolks of eggs in a bowl, add cream, beat well together, and add lobster. Gently shuffle all together over the fire for 2 minutes or until well thickened. Serve hot.

NUMBER OF SERVINGS: 2
TOTAL CARBO-CALORIES: 70
CARBO-CALORIES PER SERVING: 35

LOBSTER THERMIDOR

4 lobsters
2 tablespoons butter
1 teaspoon minced onion
¼ cup white wine
½ pound mushrooms, chopped fine
1 tablespoon tomato purée
2 cups Cream Sauce*
Grated Parmesan cheese

Boil lobsters, split in half, pick out all meat, leaving main body shell intact. Dice tail parts, coral, and claws into good-sized pieces. Heat butter in skillet. Add onion, lobster, and wine. Cook 5 minutes, stirring constantly. Add mushrooms, tomato. Cook 5 minutes more. Place mixture in shells, pour enough Cream Sauce over mixture to fill shells, sprinkle with cheese. Bake in oven, 375° F., until thoroughly heated, brown a few minutes under broiler, and serve.

NUMBER OF SERVINGS: 4
TOTAL CARBO-CALORIES: 84
CARBO-CALORIES PER SERVING: 21

FRIED OYSTERS

24 large oysters
½ cup bread crumbs
1 teaspoon salt
⅛ teaspoon pepper
1 egg, beaten
Parsley, pickle, or lemon

Clean and drain select oysters. Roll in bread crumbs seasoned with salt and pepper. Let stand 15 minutes or more, then dip in egg, roll in crumbs again, let stand again 15 minutes or more in a cool place, then fry 1 minute in deep, hot fat or until golden brown. Drain on paper, serve on hot platter with parsley, pickle, or lemon.

NUMBER OF SERVINGS: 4
TOTAL CARBO-CALORIES: 86
CARBO-CALORIES PER SERVING: 21½

OYSTERS À LA POULETTE

1 tablespoon butter
1 tablespoon flour
1 cup bouillon or oyster liquor
Salt and cayenne
Juice ½ lemon
4 egg yolks
½ pint cream
30 large oysters

Heat butter, add flour, then bouillon, and when well cooked and smooth, add seasoning, lemon juice and egg yolks beaten with the cream. Steam oysters, pour sauce over them, and cook 2 minutes.

NUMBER OF SERVINGS: 5
TOTAL CARBO-CALORIES: 140
CARBO-CALORIES PER SERVING: 28

OYSTERS AND MUSHROOMS

12 large mushrooms
12 large oysters
Salt and pepper
2 tablespoons butter
1 cup Brown Sauce*

Wash and remove stems of mushrooms. Chop stems for sauce. Sauté caps and stems separately. Place mushrooms in dripping pan, hollow side up, place an oyster on each cap, season with salt, pepper, and butter, and cook until oysters are plump. Serve with the stems in Brown Sauce.

NUMBER OF SERVINGS: 2
TOTAL CARBO-CALORIES: 76
CARBO-CALORIES PER SERVING: 38

PAN-BROILED OYSTERS

2 tablespoons butter
1/8 teaspoon white pepper
1 teaspoon salt
Cayenne
1 pint oysters
1 cup oyster liquor
1 cup hot cream

Place butter and seasoning in frying pan. When hot, add the oysters, cover, and shake pan. When oysters are nearly plump, add liquor and cream, mixed. When hot, serve.

NUMBER OF SERVINGS: 4
TOTAL CARBO-CALORIES: 76
CARBO-CALORIES PER SERVING: 19

FRIED SCALLOPS

Pick over and wash quickly 1 quart scallops. Parboil 3 minutes. Drain and dry between towels. Prepare like Fried Oysters*.

NUMBER OF SERVINGS: 4
TOTAL CARBO-CALORIES: 64
CARBO-CALORIES PER SERVING: 16

BOILED SHRIMP

1 *pound fresh shrimp*
2 *tablespoons salt*
1 *tablespoon caraway seed*

Wash shrimp. Bring 1½ quarts water to a boil, add salt and caraway seed, add shrimp, let boil 12 to 15 minutes or until tender. Let stand in liquid until cool. Drain and keep in a cool place, and when ready to serve remove shell and black line at the top. Serve hot with Cream Sauce* or prepare as Fried Oysters*, or serve cold as a salad with celery and French Dressing*.

NUMBER OF SERVINGS: 4
TOTAL CARBO-CALORIES: 24
CARBO-CALORIES PER SERVING: 6

FRIED SHRIMP

1 *pound large raw shrimp in shell*
Salt and pepper
1 *egg, slightly beaten*
1 *cup flour*
Vegetable oil or fat

Wash, rinse, and drain shrimp. Split along back, remove shell, leaving on first tail joint and tail. Take out black line at top. Place in refrigerator about 2 hours. Dip shrimp into seasoned egg, roll in flour, and fry a few at a time in deep, hot fat until light brown. Splitting allows shrimp to curl while frying. Serve hot with catsup or chili sauce.

NUMBER OF SERVINGS: 4
TOTAL CARBO-CALORIES: 128
CARBO-CALORIES PER SERVING: 32

SHRIMP WIGGLE

4 tablespoons butter
2 tablespoons flour
½ teaspoon salt
Paprika
1½ cups milk
1 cup cut-up, boiled shrimp
1 cup canned peas, drained
6 patty shells

Melt the butter and add flour, salt, and a little paprika. Pour the milk in gradually, stirring until thick. Add shrimp and peas. Heat, pour into heated patty shells, and serve.

NUMBER OF SERVINGS: 6
TOTAL CARBO-CALORIES: 90
CARBO-CALORIES PER SERVING: 15

POULTRY

CHICKEN FRICASSEE

1 chicken (3½ pounds)
½ cup each of minced onion and celery
Salt, pepper, and ginger
3 tablespoons chicken fat or butter
4 tablespoons flour
Cream Sauce*

Boil chicken with vegetables and seasoning, cook until tender; save broth. Melt fat in frying pan, add flour, stir well, and gradually pour on 2 cups chicken broth. Drain, serve with Cream Sauce.

NUMBER OF SERVINGS: 8
TOTAL CARBO-CALORIES: 220
CARBO-CALORIES PER SERVING: 27½

CHICKEN À LA KING

1 young chicken (3½ pounds)
1 green pepper
1 pimiento
2 cups White Sauce*
1 cup chicken stock
1 cup sliced mushrooms
3 tablespoons butter
¼ cup sherry
Salt, pepper, and paprika to taste
2 egg yolks, beaten

Stew the chicken, take the large white and dark pieces, cut
with scissors into thick strips 2 inches long. Cut green pepper
into thin strips, pimiento into small pieces. Make White
Sauce using cream. Add chicken stock, stirring all together
constantly until thick and smooth. Place where it will keep
hot. Sauté mushrooms and green pepper in the butter 5 minutes, stirring often. Add to the sauce. Stir in sherry gradually,
season to taste with salt, pepper, and paprika. Then add
chicken and pimiento. Let simmer a few minutes until well
heated. Just before serving, add the egg yolks with a little
water. Cook 1 minute longer.

NUMBER OF SERVINGS: 7
TOTAL CARBO-CALORIES: 210
CARBO-CALORIES PER SERVING: 30

CHICKEN PAPRIKA

   ¼ cup butter or fat
   1 chicken (3½ pounds)
   1 teaspoon salt
   ¼ cup flour
   1 teaspoon paprika

Heat fat in heavy kettle, add chicken, cut at joints, seasoned,
and rolled in flour mixed with paprika. Brown, add 1½ cups
hot water, and let cook slowly on top of stove or in oven,
well covered, 2½ hours or until tender.

NUMBER OF SERVINGS: 7
TOTAL CARBO-CALORIES: 196
CARBO-CALORIES PER SERVING: 28

CHICKEN SPANISH

1 fat chicken (4 pounds)
Salt, pepper, and paprika
¼ cup chicken fat or butter
1 Spanish onion, sliced
1 medium can tomatoes
3 carrots, chopped fine
1 celery root or stalk in small cubes
1 green pepper, seeds removed
1 small can mushrooms
1 small can peas, drained

Dress, clean, and cut the chicken in pieces to serve. Season with salt, pepper, and paprika. Heat fat, add onion, and brown; add chicken, brown lightly, and let cook very slowly in covered casserole about 1 hour. Add tomatoes, carrots, celery, and pepper, cover again, and let cook until tender. Ten minutes before serving add mushrooms and peas. Season to taste.

Number of Servings:	8
Total Carbo-calories:	336
Carbo-calories per Serving:	42

FRIED SPRING CHICKEN

1 spring chicken (1½ pounds)
Salt, pepper, and ginger
Flour
¼ cup butter or chicken fat

Season chicken with salt, pepper, and ginger. Dredge with flour and fry in plenty of butter or hot fat in a frying pan until brown. Cover, place over low flame or in slow oven for 1 hour until tender.

Number of Servings:	3
Total Carbo-calories:	102
Carbo-calories per Serving:	34

STEWED CHICKEN

Veal bone
Salt and pepper
½ cup each chopped onion and celery
1 chicken (4 pounds)

In a kettle large enough to hold the chicken, put the veal bone, seasoning, and vegetables. Cover with 3 quarts cold water. Let cook about 1 hour, then plunge the whole chicken, previously well seasoned, into the boiling broth. Cover and simmer slowly until chicken is tender.

NUMBER OF SERVINGS: 8
TOTAL CARBO-CALORIES: 200
CARBO-CALORIES PER SERVING: 25

CHICKEN CUSTARD

4 egg yolks
⅛ teaspoon salt
1 cup cream
1 cup strong chicken soup

Beat yolks until thick and lemon colored, add salt, beat into the cream; stir in the hot soup. Pour into small custard cups and bake in water in a moderate oven, 350° F.

NUMBER OF SERVINGS: 2
TOTAL CARBO-CALORIES: 44
CARBO-CALORIES PER SERVING: 22

CHICKEN TIMBALES

½ *pound raw white chicken meat*
1 *pint cream*
Salt and white pepper
5 *egg whites*
2 *tablespoons butter*
1 *cup White Sauce**

Cut fine, and then pound the chicken from which the skin and sinews have been removed. Add to this, while pounding, the pint of cream, very cold, 1 teaspoon salt, and white pepper. Press through a sieve, add the egg whites, stiffly beaten, and fill little molds which have been well buttered. Place them in saucepan of water about the depth of an inch. Cover the saucepan, put into oven 20 minutes, 375° F. Turn out of molds onto platter, serve with White Sauce.

NUMBER OF SERVINGS:	12
TOTAL CARBO-CALORIES:	120
CARBO-CALORIES PER SERVING:	10

CHICKEN LIVERS, SAUTÉED

4 *chicken livers*
½ *teaspoon salt*
⅛ *teaspoon pepper*
Flour
1 *medium onion, chopped fine*
1 *tablespoon butter*
½ *cup strong soup stock*

Cut each liver in 4 pieces, salt, pepper, and dredge well with flour. Fry onion in butter until light brown. Put in livers and shake pan over fire to sear all sides. Add soup stock. Allow to boil up once. Serve immediately.

NUMBER OF SERVINGS:	2
TOTAL CARBO-CALORIES:	50
CARBO-CALORIES PER SERVING:	25

MEATS

BEEF À LA MODE

Clove garlic
3 pounds top round
2 tablespoons beef fat
1 large onion, sliced
1 large or 2 medium carrots, chopped
2 stalks celery, chopped
2 teaspoons salt and pepper
Paprika
¾ cup tomato purée
1 thick slice rye bread

Cut clove of garlic and rub well over meat. Heat beef fat in Dutch oven or any kettle with a close-fitting cover until smoking hot. Add onion and, when slightly cooked, add meat and brown thoroughly on all sides. Add carrots, celery, and seasoning. Cover tightly and cook slowly for 2½ hours. Then add tomato purée and the bread, crumbled, and cook until done.

NUMBER OF SERVINGS:	9
TOTAL CARBO-CALORIES:	108
CARBO-CALORIES PER SERVING:	12

BEEF EN CASSEROLE

Salt and pepper to taste
2½ pounds beef, chuck or round
1 tablespoon flour
2 tablespoons beef drippings
1 small carrot, diced
1 small onion, sliced
1 cup strained tomatoes
1 bay leaf

Salt and pepper meat, cut in pieces, dust with flour. Heat fat in a frying pan and brown the meat in it on all sides. Place meat in casserole, add other ingredients, cover, and let simmer at a low temperature in oven until tender, keeping the casserole well covered so as not to allow the steam and juices to escape. Let cook 2½ hours.

NUMBER OF SERVINGS:	8
TOTAL CARBO-CALORIES:	128
CARBO-CALORIES PER SERVING:	16

BEEF STEW

3½ pounds stewing beef
¼ cup flour
Salt and pepper
2 tablespoons beef drippings
½ onion, chopped
¼ cup chopped turnips
¼ cup chopped carrots
2 potatoes
Dumplings

Wipe the meat, remove all the small pieces of bone, and cut into small pieces. Put the larger bones and tough meat into the kettle and cover with cold water. Dredge the rest of the meat with flour, salt and pepper, and brown it in the melted fat in the frying pan. Brown the onion also, then put the meat and onion into the kettle and let simmer 2 or 3 hours or until the meat is tender. Half an hour before serving add the other vegetables; 15 minutes before serving add dumplings. Cook 15 minutes. When done take out the dumplings, remove the pieces of bone and fat. If necessary, thicken the gravy with flour and add some pepper and salt.

NUMBER OF SERVINGS:	10
TOTAL CARBO-CALORIES:	235
CARBO-CALORIES PER SERVING:	23½

CHILI CON CARNE

1 cup kidney beans
½ teaspoon baking soda
1 pound fresh beef, cut in small pieces or ground
2 teaspoons fat
1 teaspoon chili powder
1 medium onion, chopped
½ cup chopped fresh tomato
½ teaspoon paprika
Salt to taste
Flour

Soak the beans overnight in cold water. Cook until tender in 1 quart fresh water to which ½ teaspoon soda has been added. Drain well. Brown the meat in the hot fat, add chili powder and onion, fry brown. Add the tomato, paprika, salt, and 1 cup water, and cook until the meat is tender. Add beans. Bring to a boil and thicken with flour. Serve hot.

NUMBER OF SERVINGS:	4
TOTAL CARBO-CALORIES:	118
CARBO-CALORIES PER SERVING:	29½

CHOPPED BEEF IN CABBAGE LEAVES

8 large cabbage leaves
1 pound lean raw beef, chopped
Salt and pepper to taste
1 teaspoon onion juice
½ cup cooked rice
2 cups tomatoes
1 onion, chopped
2 tablespoons vinegar
Artificial sweetener equivalent to 2 tablespoons sugar

Soak the cabbage leaves in hot water a few minutes to make them less brittle. Season the meat highly with salt and pepper, add onion juice and rice. Roll a portion of the meat mixture in each leaf. Place them in a kettle with the rest of the ingredients, add a little water, and let simmer until cabbage is tender and well browned.

NUMBER OF SERVINGS: 4
TOTAL CARBO-CALORIES: 74
CARBO-CALORIES PER SERVING: 18½

CHOPPED STEAK (HAMBURGER)

1 pound round steak, chopped
1 teaspoon salt
¼ teaspoon pepper

Mix ingredients lightly together with 3 tablespoons ice water and shape into small cakes, about ¾ inch thick. Grease pan or broiler with fat scraps. Brown meat and cook from 2 to 5 minutes on one side and then on the other side.

NUMBER OF SERVINGS: 3
TOTAL CARBO-CALORIES: 42
CARBO-CALORIES PER SERVING: 14

FILLET OF BEEF

Fillet of beef (4 pounds)
4 tablespoons bacon fat
Salt and pepper
¼ cup melted butter
1 tablespoon lemon juice
1 tablespoon Worcestershire sauce

Lard fillet with bacon fat. Season with salt and pepper. Cover with butter and lemon juice. Let stand several hours. Broil a few minutes, then put into hot oven, 450° F., adding Worcestershire sauce and basting often. Roast from 30 to 45 minutes. Thicken gravy in pan.

NUMBER OF SERVINGS:	12
TOTAL CARBO-CALORIES:	312
CARBO-CALORIES PER SERVING:	26

HUNGARIAN GOULASH

1 pound lean beef
1 pound lean veal
½ cup flour
1 tablespoon fat
1 large onion, diced
1 teaspoon salt
1 teaspoon paprika
1 cup strained tomatoes
4 small potatoes

Cut beef and veal into 1-inch cubes, roll in flour, and brown in hot fat with the onion, salt, and paprika. Add tomatoes. Cook 1 hour; then ½ hour before serving, add potatoes. Let cook slowly, closely covered, until potatoes are done.

NUMBER OF SERVINGS:	6
TOTAL CARBO-CALORIES:	138
CARBO-CALORIES PER SERVING:	23

ITALIAN ROLLED MEAT

1½ pounds round steak, ½ inch thick
2 tablespoons cooking fat
½ pound sliced boiled ham
¼ pound chopped beef
Salt and pepper
6 hard-cooked eggs
Oil or fat for frying
Italian Tomato Sauce*

Spread steak with fat. Lay ham evenly over steak. Spread chopped beef, well seasoned with salt and pepper, over ham. Place eggs in a row down the center. Form into one large roll and tie with string. Brown all over in hot fat. Place in sauce-pan with Italian Tomato Sauce and let cook slowly until tender. Remove string. Serve hot or cold, sliced.

NUMBER OF SERVINGS: 6
TOTAL CARBO-CALORIES: 171
CARBO-CALORIES PER SERVING: 28½

MEAT LOAF

1 pound beef
½ pound veal
Small piece suet
¼ pound bread
2 eggs
¼ cup chopped walnuts
1 teaspoon salt
Onion and celery salt
½ cup canned tomatoes
4 strips bacon
1 tablespoon fat

Run meat and fat through chopper. Soak bread in water and squeeze dry. Beat eggs well, add meat, nuts, seasoning, tomatoes, and bread. Mix thoroughly, form into loaf, lay strips of bacon on top, place in roasting pan with 1 tablespoon fat. Place in moderate oven, 350° F., for 1 hour; baste often, adding water only if necessary.

NUMBER OF SERVINGS: 6
TOTAL CARBO-CALORIES: 198
CARBO-CALORIES PER SERVING: 33

NEW ENGLAND BOILED DINNER

4 pounds corned beef
3 large carrots
2 small turnips
6 small parsnips
1 small cabbage
6 medium onions
6 medium potatoes

Wash meat in cold water. If very salty, soak ½ hour in cold water; or let come to a boil, then drain. Place meat in kettle with boiling water to cover. Let cook slowly 3 to 5 hours or until tender. Two hours before serving, add carrots, and turnips cut in quarters; and ½ hour before serving add parsnips, cabbage, onions, and potatoes. Serve attractively arranged on a large platter.

NUMBER OF SERVINGS: 12
TOTAL CARBO-CALORIES: 528
CARBO-CALORIES PER SERVING: 44

POT ROAST

Salt and pepper
2½ pounds beef, chuck, rump, or flank steak
Sprinkle flour
2 tablespoons drippings
1 onion, chopped fine
1 or 2 bay leaves
1 medium carrot
1 sliced celery root
1 cup canned tomatoes
1 tablespoon flour

Season meat and sprinkle with flour. Heat the fat and fry the onion in it until light brown; add the meat, brown on all sides to keep in the juices. Pour on 1 cup boiling water, add bay leaves, carrot, and celery root, cover tightly, then let simmer slowly about 2½ hours, or until tender. Add a little boiling water to prevent burning. About ½ hour before serving add tomatoes. Thicken gravy with flour. If closely covered kettle is used, lower flame and use less water.

NUMBER OF SERVINGS: 7
TOTAL CARBO-CALORIES: 161
CARBO-CALORIES PER SERVING: 23

RUMP ROAST

¼ pound raw beef fat in small chunks
1 clove garlic, chopped fine
Salt, pepper, and ginger
Rump of beef (3 pounds, a thick chunk)
¼ cup diced onion
¼ cup diced celery
¼ cup diced carrots
1 tablespoon flour

Mix beef fat, garlic, salt, pepper, and ginger together. Make deep gashes in the meat, about 2 inches apart, filling pockets with the fat cubes and garlic mixture, pressing the mixture in well. Put meat in kettle, pour over boiling water to cover, cover, and let cook gently 1½ hours, adding more water as needed. Add onion, celery, and carrots to soup and let cook 1 hour longer. Remove meat when tender. Season all over again with salt, pepper, and ginger. Place in roasting pan, add fat from top of soup, place in hot oven, and roast until well browned, basting often with fat in pan. Place roast on hot platter, add a little flour to gravy in roasting pan and 1 cup hot soup. Stir and cook until smooth, then pour over meat and serve.

NUMBER OF SERVINGS: 9
TOTAL CARBO-CALORIES: 225
CARBO-CALORIES PER SERVING: 25

SWEET AND SOUR BEEF

Brisket of beef (3 pounds)
Salt and pepper
A little dill
Small piece bay leaf
1 onion, sliced
Juice 1 lemon
Artificial sweetener equivalent to 3 tablespoons sugar

Place the meat in a stewpan, adding salt, pepper, dill, and bay leaf for seasoning. Add the onion, sliced thin, and 1 cup boiling water. Stew meat until tender, about 2½ hours. Add lemon juice and sweetener to taste until sweet and sour.

NUMBER OF SERVINGS: 12
TOTAL CARBO-CALORIES: 192
CARBO-CALORIES PER SERVING: 16

SWISS STEAK

3 pounds round steak, cut 1½ inches thick
1 clove garlic
¼ cup flour
2 teaspoons salt
⅛ teaspoon pepper
3 tablespoons fat
1 medium onion, sliced

Put steak on board, cut garlic in half, and rub over the meat. Pound the flour, salt, and pepper into the steak with the edge of a heavy earthen saucer or meat mallet, first on one side and then on the other. Cut into individual portions if desired. Melt fat in frying pan, add onion, let brown slightly, set to one side, put in meat, season, and let brown on both sides. Add 2 cups of boiling water, cover closely, and let simmer 2 to 3 hours, or until tender.

NUMBER OF SERVINGS: 9
TOTAL CARBO-CALORIES: 234
CARBO-CALORIES PER SERVING: 26

ROAST LEG OF LAMB

Make several incisions on each side of 3-pound leg of lamb through the skin and insert thin slice of garlic in each pocket. Salt, pepper, and dredge meat with ¼ cup flour, place in roasting pan without water, skin side down. Roast in hot oven, 480° F., for about 30 minutes. If roast is lean, brush with butter or poultry fat. When lightly browned, reduce heat to 300° F., continue cooking, uncovered without water, about 2 to 3 hours or 30 to 35 minutes a pound, depending upon age of lamb.

NUMBER OF SERVINGS: 8
TOTAL CARBO-CALORIES: 164
CARBO-CALORIES PER SERVING: 20½

STUFFED LAMB CHOPS

6 lamb chops
6 chicken livers
Salt and pepper

Have rib or loin chops cut 2 inches thick. Remove bone and outer skin. Make slit in each chop and place a chicken liver near long end, drawing end of chop around into round, flat piece with string. Place in greased broiler, under hot flame, brown on both sides. Lower rack, let broil, turning often, 15 to 20 minutes longer. Remove string, sprinkle with salt and pepper. Dot with bits of butter, remove to hot platter, and serve.

NUMBER OF SERVINGS: 8
TOTAL CARBO-CALORIES: 69
CARBO-CALORIES PER SERVING: 11½

BAKED HAM WITH APPLES OR PINEAPPLE

1 slice raw ham (2 pounds, 1 inch thick)
¼ cup brown sugar
1 teaspoon cloves
4 medium-sized tart apples or 1 cup grated pineapple

Wash and trim ham. Rub in 1 tablespoon of the sugar. Place in pan and sprinkle with cloves. Pare and cut apples in eighths, lay them around and over ham, sprinkle the remaining sugar over apples. Or, if you prefer, pour over 1 cup of grated pineapple instead of apples and sugar. Pour ½ cup water around meat. Cover and bake 1½ hours or until ham is tender. Uncover last 15 minutes.

NUMBER OF SERVINGS:	6
TOTAL CARBO-CALORIES:	267
CARBO-CALORIES PER SERVING:	44½

PORK CHOPS WITH APPLES

2 pork chops, 1½ inches thick
Salt and pepper
1 large apple, sliced ½ inch thick
1 tablespoon sugar

Sprinkle pork chops with salt and pepper. Cover each chop with half of an unpeeled apple, cut crosswise and cored, placing cut side on chop. Sprinkle apple with sugar, place in pan, in medium oven, 350° F., and bake 30 to 40 minutes, basting often, until well browned and done. Serve hot with gravy.

NUMBER OF SERVINGS:	2
TOTAL CARBO-CALORIES:	74
CARBO-CALORIES PER SERVING:	37

ROAST PORK

Rub a 3-pound roast with salt and pepper and place in roaster, fat side up, uncovered and without water. Place in oven at 500° F. for 15 to 20 minutes, or until fat is nicely browned. Reduce heat to 350° F. and allow to roast 30 to 35 minutes per pound. Or you may roast it at 350° F. the entire time. Pork must be thoroughly cooked. Baste occasionally with the fat in the pan. An onion may be placed on the roast.

NUMBER OF SERVINGS:	9
TOTAL CARBO-CALORIES:	202½
CARBO-CALORIES PER SERVING:	22½

SPARERIBS AND SAUERKRAUT

3 pounds spareribs
1½ pounds sauerkraut

Brown spareribs in skillet. Place in large kettle or Dutch oven, cover with sauerkraut, and simmer slowly for 2 hours.

NUMBER OF SERVINGS: 6
TOTAL CARBO-CALORIES: 276
CARBO-CALORIES PER SERVING: 46

BAKED VEAL CHOPS

4 veal chops, bone cut short
Salt, pepper, and flour
2 tablespoons butter
½ pint cream
Juice ½ lemon
1 egg yolk

Season chops lightly with salt and pepper. Dip in flour. Heat skillet, add butter; when hot, add chops. Fry slowly for 20 minutes, turning to brown evenly. Remove to oven. Bake 20 minutes. Mix cream and lemon juice, pour over chops, and bake 20 minutes more. Just before serving, pour sauce from pan onto well-beaten yolk mixed with a little cream.

NUMBER OF SERVINGS: 4
TOTAL CARBO-CALORIES: 128
CARBO-CALORIES PER SERVING: 32

PAPRIKA SCHNITZEL

Cut 1½ pounds veal steak in pieces for serving. Salt and pepper, roll in flour. Heat 2 tablespoons fat in skillet, add paprika until red, then 3 onions, sliced, fried until glassy. Add meat, brown all over, gradually add ½ cup thick sour cream, cover pan, let cook slowly, ½ hour or until tender. Add a little water and serve.

NUMBER OF SERVINGS:	4
TOTAL CARBO-CALORIES:	111
CARBO-CALORIES PER SERVING:	27¾

BOILED SMOKED TONGUE

1 smoked tongue (2 pounds)
6 bay leaves
1 teaspoon whole pepper
1 teaspoon cloves
1 onion, sliced

Wash the tongue and, if salty, soak in cold water overnight. Place in kettle with water to cover, seasonings, and onion, and let simmer slowly until tender, from 3 to 5 hours or until the skin curls back.

Then remove from the brine, pull off the outer skin, cut off root, and let cool in the brine. May be sliced cold or served hot.

NUMBER OF SERVINGS:	6
TOTAL CARBO-CALORIES:	105
CARBO-CALORIES PER SERVING:	17½

CALF'S HEART

Wash, remove the veins and blood clots from a 1-pound heart. Sprinkle heart with salt and pepper, dredge with ¼ cup flour, and brown all over in 2 tablespoons fat. Place in deep pan, half cover with boiling water, cover closely, and bake slowly 2 hours. Thicken liquid with flour, pour over heart.

NUMBER OF SERVINGS:	3
TOTAL CARBO-CALORIES:	63
CARBO-CALORIES PER SERVING:	21

FRIED LIVER WITH ONIONS OR BACON

Calf's liver, sliced (1 pound)
Salt and pepper
2 tablespoons flour
2 tablespoons bacon fat or butter
1 large onion, sliced, or ¼ cup bacon bits

Clean liver. Salt and pepper to taste, then dredge with the flour. Heat skillet, add the fat. Fry liver slices a few minutes on each side until brown. Reduce heat, let cook slowly about 5 minutes more for rare, 10 minutes for well done. Too-long cooking makes liver tough and dry. Serve with fried onions or bacon.

NUMBER OF SERVINGS: 3
TOTAL CARBO-CALORIES: 108
CARBO-CALORIES PER SERVING: 36

FRIED SWEETBREADS

1 pound sweetbreads
¼ cup fine bread crumbs
½ teaspoon salt
⅛ teaspoon pepper
⅛ teaspoon ginger
1 egg

Parboil sweetbreads; roll in bread crumbs and seasoning, then egg, and again in crumbs. Fry a nice brown in deep, hot fat or in the frying pan with a little fat.

NUMBER OF SERVINGS: 4
TOTAL CARBO-CALORIES: 148
CARBO-CALORIES PER SERVING: 37

HONEYCOMB TRIPE

Wash carefully 1 pound of tripe that has not been pickled, and cut into 1-inch squares. Put it into a stew pan with ¼ teaspoon each of salt, sugar, and prepared mustard, with water enough to cover (about 1 pint). Boil up and skim carefully, simmer for 3 hours, watch closely to prevent sticking, skim if necessary. Stir in 1 tablespoon flour mixed with a little cold water, simmer ½ hour longer, season well, and serve.

NUMBER OF SERVINGS: 3
TOTAL CARBO-CALORIES: 63
CARBO-CALORIES PER SERVING: 21

KIDNEYS

Plunge 1 pound of veal kidneys in boiling water, remove skins, soak in cold salted water 30 minutes. Slice kidneys, remove tubes and tissue, season with salt and pepper. Heat 2 tablespoons poultry fat, add 1 tablespoon chopped onion, fry 2 minutes, add kidneys, let cook for 5 minutes. Cover with Brown Sauce*.

NUMBER OF SERVINGS: 3
TOTAL CARBO-CALORIES: 33
CARBO-CALORIES PER SERVING: 11

POTATOES, RICE, AND PASTAS

LYONNAISE POTATOES

1 pound cold boiled potatoes
Salt and pepper
1 teaspoon chopped onion
2 tablespoons beef drippings or butter
2 tablespoons chopped parsley

Cut the potatoes into slices, season with the salt and pepper. Fry the onion in the drippings till light brown, put in the potatoes and cook until they have taken up the fat. Add parsley and serve.

NUMBER OF SERVINGS: 4
TOTAL CARBO-CALORIES: 116
CARBO-CALORIES PER SERVING: 29

MASHED POTATOES

6 medium potatoes
3 tablespoons butter
⅓ cup hot milk
1 teaspoon salt

Boil potatoes. Rub through a ricer, or mash, and add the rest of the ingredients in their order. Beat with a fork until creamy, and pile lightly on a hot dish. Keep hot over hot water until ready to serve. Dot with butter. Sprinkle with paprika.

NUMBER OF SERVINGS: 6
TOTAL CARBO-CALORIES: 144
CARBO-CALORIES PER SERVING: 24

POTATO CHARLOTTE

3 cups raw grated potatoes
2 slices wheat bread soaked in milk
2 eggs, beaten
1 tablespoon salt
1 teaspoon paprika
1 medium onion, chopped
3 tablespoons poultry fat

To grated potatoes add soaked bread, eggs, and seasoning. Fry onion in the fat and add to mixture. Heat and grease iron skillet well, pour in the mixture, bake in hot oven, 475° F., until well browned on top.

NUMBER OF SERVINGS: 4
TOTAL CARBO-CALORIES: 110
CARBO-CALORIES PER SERVING: 27½

POTATOES ON THE HALF SHELL

6 medium-sized baked potatoes
2 tablespoons butter
1 teaspoon salt
¼ cup hot milk
Melted butter
1 cup grated American cheese

Cut fresh or leftover potatoes in half lengthwise, scoop out the inside. Mash and mix with the butter, salt, and milk, and beat well. Return to the shells, brush tops with melted butter, and sprinkle with the cheese. Place in moderate oven, 350° F., bake about 5 to 10 minutes, and serve.

NUMBER OF SERVINGS:	12
TOTAL CARBO-CALORIES:	165
CARBO-CALORIES PER SERVING:	13¾

SCALLOPED POTATOES

2 pounds raw potatoes
2 tablespoons butter
Salt
2 cups White Sauce*

Wash, pare, and soak potatoes, cut into ½-inch slices. Butter a baking dish, place a layer of potatoes at the bottom, sprinkle with salt. Cover with White Sauce, then repeat. Bake 1 hour or longer, until potatoes are soft and browned over the top.

NUMBER OF SERVINGS:	10
TOTAL CARBO-CALORIES:	280
CARBO-CALORIES PER SERVING:	28

BAKED SWEET POTATOES

Select 6 even-sized sweet potatoes. Scrub. Place in a hot oven at 400° F. for ¾ hour or until done. Or parboil in boiling salted water and then bake in the oven until soft.

NUMBER OF SERVINGS:	6
TOTAL CARBO-CALORIES:	216
CARBO-CALORIES PER SERVING:	36

CURRIED RICE

1 cup rice
2 teaspoons salt
3 cups hot chicken broth
1 medium onion, chopped fine
2 tablespoons butter
2 teaspoons curry powder

Cover rice with salted cold water, bring quickly to boiling point, drain, and rinse in cold water. Then cook in the chicken broth, and when half done, add the onion sautéed in butter and the curry powder creamed with a little butter. Mix thoroughly, add more stock if needed, and finish cooking in a slow oven, 300° F.

NUMBER OF SERVINGS: 4
TOTAL CARBO-CALORIES: 118
CARBO-CALORIES PER SERVING: 29½

ITALIAN RICE
(Risotto)

2 tablespoons chicken fat
2 tablespoons chopped onion
1 teaspoon chopped parsley
¼ pound chicken livers
1 cup rice
2 teaspoons salt
3 cups hot chicken soup
⅛ teaspoon Spanish saffron
3 tablespoons grated Romano cheese

Heat fat in top of double boiler, add onion, parsley, and livers, diced. Let fry gently until well browned, stirring constantly. Add rice well cleaned, let fry until light yellow, then gradually add salted soup. Let boil well for 5 minutes, add saffron dissolved in a little hot soup and strained, stir well, cover kettle, and let cook over hot water 20 to 30 minutes or until tender. Add cheese, mix lightly, and serve hot with more grated cheese.

NUMBER OF SERVINGS: 4
TOTAL CARBO-CALORIES: 112
CARBO-CALORIES PER SERVING: 28

SPANISH RICE

1 cup rice
4 tablespoons cooking fat
2 medium onions, chopped
2 cloves garlic
2 cups tomato sauce
1 red or green pepper, chopped
2 teaspoons salt
1 teaspoon paprika

Wash rice thoroughly, place in frying pan with bacon or poultry fat, add onion and the garlic minced fine. Let fry 10 minutes, add 1 cup water and rest of the ingredients, cook slowly about 1 hour, and as water evaporates, add more to keep it from burning, until rice is tender.

NUMBER OF SERVINGS: 6
TOTAL CARBO-CALORIES: 183
CARBO-CALORIES PER SERVING: 30½

MACARONI AND CHEESE

Boil ½ pound macaroni and prepare 1 cup White Sauce*. Have ready 1 cup grated cheese. Butter a pudding dish, put in a layer of macaroni, one of sauce, and one of cheese, then another layer of each, with cheese on top. Dust the top with sifted bread or cracker crumbs, dot with bits of butter, and bake 15 minutes in a hot oven, 425° F. Serve in dish.

NUMBER OF SERVINGS: 4
TOTAL CARBO-CALORIES: 152
CARBO-CALORIES PER SERVING: 38

MACARONI AND OYSTERS

1 pint oysters
1 pint boiled macaroni
1 cup White Sauce*
½ cup crackers, rolled
2 tablespoons butter

Into a well-greased pudding dish place drained oysters and macaroni, cover with White Sauce which has some of the oyster liquor in it. Sprinkle with cracker crumbs and bits of butter. Bake until browned.

NUMBER OF SERVINGS: 5
TOTAL CARBO-CALORIES: 200
CARBO-CALORIES PER SERVING: 40

SPAGHETTI ITALIENNE

½ pound spaghetti
1 medium can tomatoes
2 cloves garlic, cut fine
4 bay leaves
¼ teaspoon pepper
¼ cup olive oil
Salt to taste
¼ cup grated Parmesan cheese

Boil spaghetti in 2 quarts of water. Drain the tomatoes (set aside the pulp for some future use), and place liquid tomato in saucepan with the garlic, bay leaves, pepper, and oil. Salt to taste. Cook until well seasoned, strain, and pour over the spaghetti. Serve, sprinkled with grated cheese.

NUMBER OF SERVINGS: 4
TOTAL CARBO-CALORIES: 116
CARBO-CALORIES PER SERVING: 29

VEGETABLES

BOILED ARTICHOKES

4 *medium artichokes*
3 *tablespoons salt*
2 *tablespoons vinegar*
4 *quarts boiling water*

With a sharp knife cut off the points of the artichokes about
1½ inches. Add salt and vinegar to 4 quarts boiling water.
Cook artichokes 20 to 30 minutes, or until leaves pull out
easily. Drain from liquid, cut each artichoke in half, lengthwise, or serve whole, removing the white fuzzy fiber or
"choke." Serve cold with French Salad Dressing* or
Vinaigrette Dressing* or Tartar Sauce*. Serve hot with
melted butter or Hollandaise Sauce*.

NUMBER OF SERVINGS: 4
TOTAL CARBO-CALORIES: 24
CARBO-CALORIES PER SERVING: 6

ASPARAGUS RING

2 *cans asparagus tips*
3 *tablespoons butter*
3 *tablespoons flour*
½ *teaspoon salt*
Pepper
1 *cup milk*
3 *eggs, separated*

Cut the asparagus into 1-inch pieces. Heat the butter, add the flour, salt, and a little pepper, stir until well blended, add ⅓ of the milk, another ⅓, then the rest, stirring until smooth. Pour this sauce onto well-beaten yolks. Cool, fold in the stiffly beaten whites of eggs and, lastly, the asparagus pieces. Place in a well-greased ring mold, set in a pan of boiling water, and bake in a moderate oven ½ hour or until set. Remove to hot platter.

NUMBER OF SERVINGS: 8
TOTAL CARBO-CALORIES: 72
CARBO-CALORIES PER SERVING: 9

BAKED BEANS

1 quart navy beans
½ pound fat salt pork or 1½ pounds brisket of beef
½ tablespoon mustard
1 tablespoon salt
2 tablespoons molasses
Artificial sweetener equivalent to 3 tablespoons sugar
1 cup boiling water

Wash, pick over beans, cover with cold water, and let soak overnight. In the morning, cover with fresh water, heat slowly, and let cook just below the boiling point until the skins burst, which is best determined by taking a few on the tip of the spoon and blowing over them; if done, the skins will burst. When done, drain beans and put in pot with the brisket of beef. If pork is used, scald it, cut through rind in ½-inch strips, bury in beans, leaving rind exposed. Mix mustard, salt, molasses, sweetener, and 1 cup boiling water, and pour over beans; add enough more water to cover them. Cover pot and bake slowly at 300° F. 6 to 8 hours. Uncover pot the last hour so that meat will brown and be crisp.

NUMBER OF SERVINGS: 12
TOTAL CARBO-CALORIES: 402
CARBO-CALORIES PER SERVING: 33½

SWEET AND SOUR BEANS

1 *quart green or wax beans*
1 *teaspoon salt*
2 *tablespoons butter*
1 *tablespoon flour*
Artificial sweetener equivalent to 2 tablespoons sugar
2 *tablespoons vinegar or lemon juice*
Salt and pepper to taste

Wash, string, and cut beans into pieces. Cook in boiling water ½ hour or until tender. Add salt when nearly done. Drain and reserve 1 cup of the bean water for the following sauce: Melt butter, add flour; then the bean liquid or soup stock and bean water mixed; then the rest of the ingredients to taste. Add the boiled beans and serve hot.

NUMBER OF SERVINGS: 8
TOTAL CARBO-CALORIES: 56
CARBO-CALORIES PER SERVING: 7

HARVARD BEETS

2 *tablespoons butter*
1 *tablespoon flour*
Artificial sweetener equivalent to ½ cup sugar
½ *teaspoon salt*
¼ *cup vinegar mixed with ¼ cup water or beet juice*
2 *cups boiled or drained canned beets*

Melt butter in saucepan or double boiler. Add flour. Stir. Add sweetener, salt, and the liquid gradually. Cook until clear, stirring constantly. Add beets and heat thoroughly.

NUMBER OF SERVINGS: 4
TOTAL CARBO-CALORIES: 34
CARBO-CALORIES PER SERVING: 8½

SAUCED BRUSSELS SPROUTS

1 quart Brussels sprouts
*1 cup White Sauce**

Pick the wilted leaves from the sprouts, cut the stalk close to the head, and soak in cold salted water 10 minutes. Drain well and cook in a large amount of rapidly boiling salted water in an open kettle only until tender. Drain and serve in White Sauce.

NUMBER OF SERVINGS: 8
TOTAL CARBO-CALORIES: 44
CARBO-CALORIES PER SERVING: 5½

CABBAGE AU GRATIN

½ large cooked cabbage
¾ cup grated American cheese
Salt and paprika
*1 pint White Sauce**
½ cup cracker crumbs
3 tablespoons melted butter

Put a layer of the cabbage, coarse-chopped, into a buttered baking dish, sprinkle with grated cheese, salt, and paprika as needed, and cover with a layer of White Sauce. Repeat the layers until all the ingredients have been used. Cover with cracker crumbs mixed with the butter. Place in oven, 350° F., until hot and the crumbs are well browned.

NUMBER OF SERVINGS: 8
TOTAL CARBO-CALORIES: 172
CARBO-CALORIES PER SERVING: 21½

CABBAGE AND SAUSAGES

6 sausages
1 quart minced cabbage
½ teaspoon pepper
Salt if necessary

Fry the sausages crisp and brown. Take from the frying pan and pour off all but 3 tablespoons of the fat. Put cabbage in frying pan with seasoning, cook until tender. Arrange in a hot dish and garnish with the sausages.

NUMBER OF SERVINGS:	4
TOTAL CARBO-CALORIES:	40
CARBO-CALORIES PER SERVING:	10

RED CABBAGE WITH CHESTNUTS

1 small red cabbage
¼ cup vinegar
2 tablespoons fat
Salt and pepper
Artificial sweetener equivalent to 1 tablespoon sugar
¼ cup raisins
1 cup chestnuts, blanched
1 tablespoon flour

Cut cabbage in fine shreds, place in colander, place colander in pan, pour 1 cup boiling water with vinegar over cabbage, let stand over pan 10 minutes. Heat fat in kettle, add cabbage seasoned with salt and pepper, let brown well, then cover and let simmer 10 minutes. To water add sweetener, raisins, and chestnuts, and let cook until chestnuts are tender. Sprinkle flour over cabbage, add to chestnuts, cook a few minutes, and serve hot.

NUMBER OF SERVINGS:	4
TOTAL CARBO-CALORIES:	102
CARBO-CALORIES PER SERVING:	25½

SPECIAL CARROTS

8 medium carrots
2 tablespoons butter or fat
2 tablespoons flour
1 cup carrot liquid

Wash, scrape carrots, cut lengthwise or crosswise, cover with 1 quart boiling salted water and cook only until tender. Make Brown Sauce* of remaining ingredients, using 1 cup of hot carrot liquid.

NUMBER OF SERVINGS: 8
TOTAL CARBO-CALORIES: 72
CARBO-CALORIES PER SERVING: 9

STEWED CELERY

1 bunch celery
*1 cup White Sauce**

Wash, scrape, and cut the outer stalks of the celery into pieces 1½ inches long. Cook in 1 quart boiling salted water only until tender. Drain and serve with White Sauce.

NUMBER OF SERVINGS: 6
TOTAL CARBO-CALORIES: 57
CARBO-CALORIES PER SERVING: 9½

BAKED EGGPLANT

Eggplant
2 tablespoons butter or fat
¼ onion, cut fine
2 tablespoons bread crumbs
Salt and pepper
1 egg yolk

Parboil eggplant until tender, but not soft, in boiling, salted water. Cut in half lengthwise with a sharp knife. Scrape out the inside and do not break the skin. Heat 1 tablespoon butter or fat, add the onion, brown, then mashed eggplant, bread crumbs, salt and pepper to taste, and the egg yolk. Mix well together, refill shells, place in pan in oven, 350° F.— baste with butter often and brown nicely.

NUMBER OF SERVINGS: 2
TOTAL CARBO-CALORIES: 60
CARBO-CALORIES PER SERVING: 30

WILTED LETTUCE

¾ pound leaf lettuce
Bacon Salad Dressing*

Wash, drain, and shred lettuce. Pour boiling water over it. Let stand 5 minutes until slightly wilted. Then drain well. Add Bacon Salad Dressing.

NUMBER OF SERVINGS: 3
TOTAL CARBO-CALORIES: 24
CARBO-CALORIES PER SERVING: 8

MACÉDOINE

1 large carrot
2 white turnips
1 pint peas
1 pint string beans
Brown Sauce*

Scrape the carrot, cut into cubes; pare the turnips and cut into cubes; put these in unsalted water and boil gently for ¾ hour, or until tender, and drain. Drain, wash, and cook the peas and beans, and add them to the vegetables; reheat over water, and use with Brown Sauce as a garnish for braised or stewed meats.

NUMBER OF SERVINGS: 8
TOTAL CARBO-CALORIES: 84
CARBO-CALORIES PER SERVING: 10½

BROILED MUSHROOMS

12 *large mushrooms*
2 *tablespoons butter*
¼ *teaspoon salt*
⅛ *teaspoon pepper*

Wash, brush fine large mushrooms, remove stems. Place caps in a buttered broiler and broil 5 minutes, under side down during first half of broiling, then turn. Put a small piece of butter in each cap, sprinkle with salt and pepper, and serve as soon as butter is melted. Keep mushrooms under side up, to keep in the juices.

NUMBER OF SERVINGS: 3
TOTAL CARBO-CALORIES: 21
CARBO-CALORIES PER SERVING: 7

CREAMED MUSHROOMS

⅔ *cup chopped mushrooms*
1½ *teaspoons butter*
1 *tablespoon cream*
1 *egg yolk*
Salt

Sauté the mushrooms in the butter. Heat the cream and egg yolk over hot water until mixture coats the spoon; add to mushrooms, and salt to taste. Serve at once.

NUMBER OF SERVINGS: 1
TOTAL CARBO-CALORIES: 11
CARBO-CALORIES PER SERVING: 11

MUSHROOMS AND SOUR CREAM

1 *pound mushrooms*
3 *tablespoons butter*
1 *cup sour cream*
Salt and paprika to taste

Wash and peel mushrooms. Place butter and 2 tablespoons water in skillet, and sauté mushrooms, turning carefully. When tender (about 15 minutes), add sour cream. Cook slowly, stirring occasionally, until sauce is of desired consistency (about 10 minutes). Season with salt and paprika.

NUMBER OF SERVINGS: 4
TOTAL CARBO-CALORIES: 48
CARBO-CALORIES PER SERVING: 12

MUSHROOM RING OR SOUFFLÉ WITH BRUSSELS SPROUTS

1 pound mushrooms
2 tablespoons butter
4 tablespoons flour
1 cup cream
4 egg yolks
4 egg whites, beaten stiff
2 cups Brussels sprouts

Chop mushrooms fine, sauté in butter until cooked. Blend flour and cream until smooth, cook until thick; pour gradually into yolks until the mixture coats the spoon; then fold in beaten whites and mushrooms. Pour into a well-buttered ring mold and set into a pan of water; bake uncovered in moderate oven, 350° F., 20 to 30 minutes. Fill center with Brussels sprouts.

NUMBER OF SERVINGS: 8
TOTAL CARBO-CALORIES: 102
CARBO-CALORIES PER SERVING: 12¾

ONIONS AND APPLES

¼ cup fat
2 pints sliced onions
8 small apples
2 teaspoons salt
Artificial sweetener to taste

Heat fat, add onions, peeled and sliced crosswise, ⅛ inch thick, and the apples, cut in quarters, pared, and cored. Cover and let steam 10 minutes, stirring occasionally until apples are soft and onions tender and slightly browned. Season with salt, and, if desired, a little sweetener. Serve hot as a vegetable.

NUMBER OF SERVINGS: 8
TOTAL CARBO-CALORIES: 128
CARBO-CALORIES PER SERVING: 16

FRENCH-FRIED ONION RINGS

Cut 1 pound of Bermuda onions in ¼-inch slices, crosswise; separate into rings. Soak in ice-cold milk for ½ hour, drain, and dry on towel. Then dredge with flour and fry, a few at a time, until brown and crisp, in deep, hot fat. Remove and drain on brown paper.

NUMBER OF SERVINGS: 8
TOTAL CARBO-CALORIES: 64
CARBO-CALORIES PER SERVING: 8

GREEN PEAS AND RICE

3 pounds fresh green peas or 1 large can peas
¼ cup butter or other fat
1 cup well-washed rice
½ teaspoon salt
Artificial sweetener equivalent to 2 tablespoons sugar

Shell the peas and wash them well; if canned peas are used, add the liquid from the can to the water in which rice is to cook. Heat the butter in a skillet, add the rice, and let simmer, stirring constantly, until rice is yellow. Add 1 quart boiling water, then the peas and seasoning. Place in pudding dish, set in the oven, and bake until rice is tender and every kernel stands out separately. Serve hot.

NUMBER OF SERVINGS: 8
TOTAL CARBO-CALORIES: 148
CARBO-CALORIES PER SERVING: 18½

STUFFED PEPPERS WITH BEEF

8 green peppers
1 pound lean raw beef, ground
1 egg
Salt and pepper
½ teaspoon onion juice
1 medium onion

Cut off stem end and remove seeds from green peppers, boil 2 minutes, drain. Mix meat with egg, salt and pepper, and onion juice. Fill peppers with meat mixture. Slice onion in a stewpan, cover slightly with water, and stew the peppers in it until well done.

NUMBER OF SERVINGS: 8
TOTAL CARBO-CALORIES: 68
CARBO-CALORIES PER SERVING: 8½

SAUERKRAUT SUPREME

2 tablespoons fat
1 medium onion, diced
1 quart sauerkraut
1 medium raw potato, grated
1 teaspoon caraway seed
Boiling water or soup stock

Heat the fat, add onion, let fry until glassy, add sauerkraut, fry 5 minutes, add potato and caraway seed, cover with boiling water or soup, cook slowly ½ hour, cover well, cook ½ hour longer on top of stove or in oven.

NUMBER OF SERVINGS: 8
TOTAL CARBO-CALORIES: 72
CARBO-CALORIES PER SERVING: 9

SPINACH PRIDE

2 pounds spinach
2 tablespoons butter or fat
1 teaspoon grated onion
2 tablespoons bread crumbs or browned flour
½ teaspoon salt
⅛ teaspoon pepper
$\frac{1}{16}$ teaspoon nutmeg
1 cup soup stock or meat gravy and hot water
1 hard-cooked egg

Pick off the roots and the decayed leaves from spinach, wash often enough to remove all sand. Put the spinach in an open kettle with a large amount of rapidly boiling salted water and cook 4 or 5 minutes, only until tender. Drain, put through food grinder or chop very fine. Heat the butter in a skillet, add the onion, then the bread crumbs or flour and the seasonings, and gradually the soup stock, spinach water, or meat gravy diluted with spinach water, then add the chopped spinach. Reheat and garnish with egg, sliced.

NUMBER OF SERVINGS: 8
TOTAL CARBO-CALORIES: 48
CARBO-CALORIES PER SERVING: 6

STUFFED SQUASH

3 large summer squash
2 tablespoons butter or fat
½ medium onion, chopped
½ cup bread soaked in water
½ teaspoon salt
⅛ teaspoon pepper
1 egg
½ cup cracker crumbs

Bake squash. Scrape out shells, being careful not to break them. Heat butter or fat in a skillet, add the onion, chopped fine, let brown lightly, add the soaked bread and the squash, mashed. Cook all together 15 minutes, stirring occasionally. Remove from fire, add the salt and pepper, and stir in the egg. Place back in shells; sprinkle cracker crumbs and bits of butter on top, return to oven to brown nicely.

NUMBER OF SERVINGS: 6
TOTAL CARBO-CALORIES: 126
CARBO-CALORIES PER SERVING: 21

SUCCOTASH

1 *cup boiled corn*
1 *cup boiled lima beans*
1 *tablespoon butter*
Salt
Pepper
¼ *cup milk*

Heat all ingredients together a few minutes and then serve.

NUMBER OF SERVINGS: 4
TOTAL CARBO-CALORIES: 98
CARBO-CALORIES PER SERVING: 24½

BROILED TOMATOES

Wash but do not peel 2 medium-sized, sound tomatoes. Cut crosswise into halves. Dip cut side into ½ cup grated, seasoned bread crumbs. Dot each half with butter. Broil only a few minutes.

NUMBER OF SERVINGS: 4
TOTAL CARBO-CALORIES: 56
CARBO-CALORIES PER SERVING: 14

VEGETARIAN LOAF

1 cup dried peas, boiled
¾ cup dried bread crumbs
¼ cup chopped walnuts
1 egg
1 teaspoon salt
⅛ teaspoon pepper
2 tablespoons melted butter
¾ cup milk

Drain peas and rub through strainer. Add other ingredients, mix well, and put in a small buttered bread pan. Cover with paper and bake 40 minutes in a slow oven, 300° F.

NUMBER OF SERVINGS: 6
TOTAL CARBO-CALORIES: 120
CARBO-CALORIES PER SERVING: 20

FRUITS

AMBROSIA

Cut a pineapple in 1-inch slices, then pare, twist off pieces to the core with strong fork. Pare 2 oranges and 1 grapefruit, separate into sections, removing membrane between. Add artificial sweetener equivalent to 1 cup sugar and juice of a lemon; place in refrigerator several hours. When ready to serve, mix with ½ cup fresh grated coconut.

NUMBER OF SERVINGS:	8
TOTAL CARBO-CALORIES:	140
CARBO-CALORIES PER SERVING:	17½

BAKED APPLES

Wash and core cooking apples. Leave peel on, or cut off ⅓ of skin at the top, or cut a strip ½ inch wide around center of apple. Place in baking dish, fill center of each apple with artificial sweetener equivalent to 1 tablespoon sugar, sprinkle with cinnamon, place 1 teaspoon butter on each apple, and cover bottom of pan with cold water. Cover pan, place in hot oven, 375° F., and bake 40 to 60 minutes, or until tender but not broken.

NUMBER OF SERVINGS:	1
TOTAL CARBO-CALORIES:	20
CARBO-CALORIES PER SERVING:	20

STEWED APRICOTS AND PRUNES

¼ pound dried apricots
¼ pound dried prunes
Artificial sweetener equivalent to ½ cup sugar
Little cinnamon

Pick over and wash the fruit. Let soak in cold water 1 hour. Put in kettle, bring to the boiling point, add sweetener and cinnamon. Let simmer until tender. Any other dried fruit may be prepared the same way.

Number of Servings: 6
Total Carbo-calories: 114
Carbo-calories per Serving: 19

BAKED BANANAS

Peel 4 bananas. Arrange in shallow baking dish, sprinkle with lemon juice. Bake in a moderate oven, 375° F., 10 to 15 minutes. Sprinkle with powdered sugar, and serve hot.

Number of Servings: 4
Total Carbo-calories: 104
Carbo-calories per Serving: 26

BROILED GRAPEFRUIT

Cut grapefruit in half, crosswise; cut out center core; loosen sections. Cover each half with ½ tablespoon butter and artificial sweetener equivalent to 2 tablespoons sugar. Broil 35 minutes at 275° F., 3½ inches from flame. Serve hot.

Number of Servings: 2
Total Carbo-calories: 32
Carbo-calories per Serving: 16

BAKED ORANGES

Grate entire rind of orange slightly. Boil 30 minutes; then cool. Cut slice off blossom end; remove core. Fill each orange with 1 teaspoon butter and artificial sweetener equivalent to 1 tablespoon sugar. Place in covered casserole filled about ⅔ full of boiling water. Bake at 275° F. for 1½ hours. Remove oranges and serve hot or cold.

NUMBER OF SERVINGS:	1
TOTAL CARBO-CALORIES:	21
CARBO-CALORIES PER SERVING:	21

BAKED PEARS

Scrub 4 medium pears. Remove blossom end. Place in round baking pan, close together, stem end up. For each pear, allow 1 tablespoon boiling water, 1 teaspoon butter, artificial sweetener equivalent to 1 tablespoon sugar. Pour around pears. Cover. Bake 1 to 2 hours in moderate oven, 375° F., depending on variety of pear. Baste occasionally.

NUMBER OF SERVINGS:	4
TOTAL CARBO-CALORIES:	108
CARBO-CALORIES PER SERVING:	27

FRIED PINEAPPLE

Take 4 ounces canned pineapple and drain. Dip pineapple in ¼ cup flour. Fry quickly on both sides in 2 tablespoons butter until delicately browned.

NUMBER OF SERVINGS:	4
TOTAL CARBO-CALORIES:	36
CARBO-CALORIES PER SERVING:	9

DESSERTS

ALMOND CAKES

⅔ cup almonds
1 tablespoon vinegar
2 tablespoons butter
5 eggs, separated
⅓ teaspoon baking powder
Pinch salt

Blanch almonds, bake until light brown, grind. Place in strainer, pour over 2 tablespoons cold water mixed with 1 tablespoon vinegar, drain. Dry in oven. Grind again. Add melted butter, yolks of eggs beaten well, baking powder, and salt. Fold in whites beaten stiff. Fill buttered gem pans ⅔ full, bake 25 minutes in slow oven, 300° F.

NUMBER OF SERVINGS: 9
TOTAL CARBO-CALORIES: 74¼
CARBO-CALORIES PER SERVING: 8¼

APPLE DELIGHT

1 egg, separated
9 almonds, blanched and chopped
⅔ cup chopped apple
Artificial sweetener equivalent to 1 teaspoon sugar
Pinch cinnamon
A little lemon rind
¾ teaspoon butter
2 teaspoons rusk crumbs

Add well-beaten egg yolk and almonds to the apple. Flavo
with sweetener, cinnamon, and lemon rind; add stiffly beaten
egg white. Grease a small shallow tin with the butter, dredge
with rusk crumbs, put in the apple mixture, and bake at
350° F.

NUMBER OF SERVINGS:	2
TOTAL CARBO-CALORIES:	33
CARBO-CALORIES PER SERVING:	16½

APPLE DESSERT

> 2½ pounds apples
> 5 eggs, separated
> Artificial sweetener equivalent to ¾ cup sugar
> 25 chopped almonds
> ¼ cup currants
> 1 tablespoon brandy
> ⅛ teaspoon cinnamon

Grate the apples. Beat egg yolks with sweetener until light,
add the apples, then the rest of the ingredients, the beaten
whites last. Place in springform and bake in moderate oven
until well set.

NUMBER OF SERVINGS:	12
TOTAL CARBO-CALORIES:	120
CARBO-CALORIES PER SERVING:	10

BLANC MANGE

> ¼ cup cornstarch
> Artificial sweetener equivalent to 2 tablespoons sugar
> ⅛ teaspoon salt
> ¼ cup cold milk
> 2 cups scalded milk
> ½ teaspoon vanilla
> 2 egg whites

Mix cornstarch, sweetener, and salt. Dilute with cold milk. Add to scalded milk and place in double boiler. Cook 15 minutes, stirring constantly until mixture thickens, and occasionally afterwards. Cool slightly. Add vanilla and stiffly beaten egg whites. Mix thoroughly, mold, and chill. Serve with a thin fruit or rum sauce if desired.

NUMBER OF SERVINGS: 5
TOTAL CARBO-CALORIES: 60
CARBO-CALORIES PER SERVING: 12

BREAD PUDDING

2 cups day-old bread cubes, crusts removed
1 teaspoon baking soda
1 cup buttermilk
Artificial sweetener equivalent to ⅓ cup sugar
1 egg
1 teaspoon mixed cinnamon, mace, cloves, and nutmeg
½ cup seedless raisins
1 tablespoon butter

Sprinkle bread cubes with soda; pour over buttermilk. Let stand until soaked. Mix well with rest of the ingredients except butter. Melt butter in top of double boiler, grease well all around. Pour mixture in and let steam 1½ hours.

NUMBER OF SERVINGS: 8
TOTAL CARBO-CALORIES: 212
CARBO-CALORIES PER SERVING: 26½

COCONUT PUDDING

1 cup bread crumbs
1 quart hot milk
1 cup grated coconut
2 tablespoons melted butter
2 eggs, slightly beaten
Artificial sweetener equivalent to 4 tablespoons sugar
Little salt
Grated rind ½ lemon

Soak the crumbs in 1 cup of the milk and mash well. Soak the coconut in the rest of the hot milk for 1 hour. Mix all together with the rest of the ingredients. Place in pudding dish and bake in a moderate oven, 350° F., until well set and brown.

NUMBER OF SERVINGS: 8
TOTAL CARBO-CALORIES: 200
CARBO-CALORIES PER SERVING: 25

COFFEE CREAM

¼ cup strong coffee
1 egg yolk, beaten
1 teaspoon gelatin
Pinch salt
Artificial sweetener equivalent to 1 teaspoon sugar
1 egg white
3½ tablespoons cream
½ teaspoon vanilla

Heat coffee, pour gradually on the egg yolk, cook until thick, stirring occasionally. Add gelatin dissolved in 2 tablespoons cold water. Add salt. Cool. Add sweetener, then the egg white, and lastly the cream stiffly beaten, flavored with vanilla. Mold and chill.

NUMBER OF SERVINGS: 1
TOTAL CARBO-CALORIES: 9½
CARBO-CALORIES PER SERVING: 9½

COFFEE CUSTARD

2 cups very hot milk
3 tablespoons ground coffee
3 eggs, beaten slightly
Artificial sweetener equivalent to 4 tablespoons sugar
¼ teaspoon vanilla

Pour milk over coffee, let steep 10 minutes, strain. Stir eggs with sweetener, add the rest. Mix, pour into small cups, and place cups in a shallow pan. Put boiling hot water in the pan until it reaches halfway up the cups. Set in a moderate oven, 350° F., and cook, until the custard is firm. Serve ice cold.

NUMBER OF SERVINGS: 4
TOTAL CARBO-CALORIES: 46
CARBO-CALORIES PER SERVING: 11½

CUP CUSTARD

2 eggs
Pinch salt
Artificial sweetener equivalent to 4 tablespoons sugar
1 pint hot milk

Beat eggs slightly, add salt and sweetener and stir, pour milk gradually into eggs. If desired, a little nutmeg or ½ teaspoon flavoring may be added. Pour into buttered cups or a pudding dish, place the cups in a pan of hot water, put the pan in a moderate oven, 325° F., and bake 30 to 45 minutes until the custards are firm in the center. Test with a knife; if the knife, inserted, comes out clean, the custard is done.

NUMBER OF SERVINGS: 4
TOTAL CARBO-CALORIES: 38
CARBO-CALORIES PER SERVING: 9½

INDIVIDUAL DELICATE CAKES

½ cup milk
2 tablespoons butter
Artificial sweetener equivalent to 1 cup sugar
1 cup flour
1 teaspoon baking powder
¼ teaspoon salt
4 egg whites
½ teaspoon cream of tartar
Vanilla or almond extract

Heat milk and butter to scalding point. Add sweetener and stir. Add flour sifted with baking powder and salt and mix thoroughly. Beat egg whites until foamy, add cream of tartar, beat until they stand up in peaks but are not dry. Fold into batter and add flavoring. Pour into greased and floured muffin tins and bake for about 25 minutes at 350° F.

Number of Servings:　　　　20
Total Carbo-calories:　　　　110
Carbo-calories per Serving:　　5½

FARINA PUDDING

¼ cup farina
1 pint scalded milk
1 tablespoon butter
Artificial sweetener equivalent to ½ cup sugar
Salt
5 eggs, separated
Lemon rind

Pour farina into scalded milk, add butter, sweetener, and salt and cook for 5 minutes. When cool, add yolks of 5 eggs, lemon rind, and whites of eggs, beaten stiff. Bake, 325° F., about 20 minutes in a pudding dish and serve at once.

Number of Servings:　　　　6
Total Carbo-calories:　　　　57
Carbo-calories per Serving:　　9½

TAPIOCA CREAM

⅓ cup quick tapioca
1 pint milk
2 eggs, separated
¼ teaspoon salt
Artificial sweetener equivalent to ⅓ cup sugar
1 teaspoon vanilla

Add tapioca to the milk and cook in double boiler until the tapioca is clear. Beat the egg yolks, add the salt and sweetener and the hot milk mixture, and cook until it thickens like soft custard. Remove from the fire, cool, fold in the whites of the eggs, beaten stiff. Flavor when cold.

NUMBER OF SERVINGS: 4
TOTAL CARBO-CALORIES: 82
CARBO-CALORIES PER SERVING: 20½

WINE SYLLABUB

Artificial sweetener equivalent to ¾ cup sugar
Juice 1 lemon
1 cup sherry or Madeira
1 pint cream
Grating of nutmeg
A little cinnamon

Mix sweetener with lemon juice and wine, add the cream, and whip to a froth. Strain if necessary. Serve very cold in glasses with nutmeg and cinnamon on top.

NUMBER OF SERVINGS: 4
TOTAL CARBO-CALORIES: 64
CARBO-CALORIES PER SERVING: 16

SANDWICHES

HOT BACON AND PEANUT BUTTER SANDWICHES

Use 1 slice wheat bread. Toast on one side. Spread thick on untoasted side with peanut butter. Sprinkle top with bacon which has been fried crisp and crumbled. Before serving, put under broiler.

NUMBER OF SERVINGS: 1
TOTAL CARBO-CALORIES: 30
CARBO-CALORIES PER SERVING: 30

CHEESE AND ANCHOVY SANDWICH

2 tablespoons butter
¼ cup grated American cheese
2 teaspoons anchovy paste
1 teaspoon vinegar
Salt, paprika, mustard to taste
2 thin slices white bread

Cream the butter, add the cheese, anchovy, and vinegar. Season and spread between slices of bread.

NUMBER OF SERVINGS: 1
TOTAL CARBO-CALORIES: 34
CARBO-CALORIES PER SERVING: 34

CHEESE, TOMATO, AND BACON SANDWICH

Cut a large round of white bread, and toast on one side. Cover untoasted side with sliced American cheese. On top of this, place ¼-inch slice of tomato and 2 slices of bacon, placed crisscross on tomato. Broil until bacon is crisp and brown.

NUMBER OF SERVINGS: 1
TOTAL CARBO-CALORIES: 13
CARBO-CALORIES PER SERVING: 13

CRAB MEAT SANDWICHES

2 hard-cooked egg yolks
1 tablespoon melted butter
1 tablespoon lemon juice
8 ounces canned crab meat
6 thin slices brown bread

Mash the egg yolks to a smooth paste with the butter, add the lemon juice and the crab, chopped fine. Mix well and spread between thin slices of bread.

NUMBER OF SERVINGS: 3
TOTAL CARBO-CALORIES: 78
CARBO-CALORIES PER SERVING: 26

EGG AND SARDINE SANDWICHES

Take 2 hard-cooked egg yolks and 1 small can of sardines, drained, skinned, and boned. Season with salt, cayenne, and mustard. Rub until smooth and add 1 teaspoon lemon juice and olive oil to make a paste. Spread on thin slices of buttered bread.

NUMBER OF SERVINGS: 2
TOTAL CARBO-CALORIES: 46
CARBO-CALORIES PER SERVING: 23

HOT HAM SANDWICH

½ pound cold boiled ham
Prepared English mustard
8 slices day-old bread
2 eggs
¾ cup milk
2 tablespoons butter

Chop the ham very fine, or put through meat grinder, and moisten thoroughly with the prepared mustard. Spread a layer of this mixture between thin slices of bread and press firmly together. Beat the eggs slightly, add milk, and beat again. Dip sandwich in this egg mixture and sauté in butter in frying pan until a golden brown on both sides. Cut the sandwiches diagonally.

NUMBER OF SERVINGS: 4
TOTAL CARBO-CALORIES: 130
CARBO-CALORIES PER SERVING: 32½

HORSERADISH SANDWICHES

Cream ¼ cup butter gradually with ¼ cup grated horse-radish, add 1 teaspoon lemon juice, a little salt, and artificial sweetener. Use 4 thin slices of rye or wheat bread and spread mixture on slices.

NUMBER OF SERVINGS: 4
TOTAL CARBO-CALORIES: 88
CARBO-CALORIES PER SERVING: 22

MIDWEST SANDWICH

Butter 2 slices of thin white bread. Trim off crusts. Place a slice of white chicken meat on 1 piece of bread. Sprinkle with Roquefort cheese. Season with paprika. Cover with the other slice, toast on both sides. Garnish with parsley; serve hot.

Number of Servings: 1
Total Carbo-calories: 28
Carbo-calories per Serving: 28

HOT MUSHROOM SANDWICHES

Sauté 1 pound mushrooms, then chop fine. Add ¾ cup White Sauce*. Spread between thin slices of bread. Press firmly together, cut in half crosswise and toast until slightly browned.

Number of Servings: 8
Total Carbo-calories: 272
Carbo-calories per Serving: 34

SHRIMP AND CHICKEN LIVER SANDWICHES

Grind ½ cup each of cooked shrimps and chicken livers, ½ Bermuda onion, and ½ green pepper, seeds removed. Season with salt, moisten with catsup or mayonnaise. Spread between thin slices of buttered bread.

Number of Servings: 3
Total Carbo-calories: 90
Carbo-calories per Serving: 30

BEVERAGES

COCOA

1 cup milk
2 teaspoons cocoa
Artificial sweetener equivalent to 2 teaspoons sugar

Scald the milk. In a saucepan put the cocoa, sweetener, and 1 cup boiling water. Boil 1 minute, then add it to the scalded milk. Taste, and add more sweetener if needed.

NUMBER OF SERVINGS: 2
TOTAL CARBO-CALORIES: 20
CARBO-CALORIES PER SERVING: 10

ICED COFFOLATE

1 tablespoon cornstarch
2 squares chocolate
½ teaspoon cinnamon
Artificial sweetener equivalent to ½ cup sugar
2 cups boiling black coffee
2 cups scalding milk

Dissolve cornstarch in a little cold water or coffee and place in double boiler with chocolate, cinnamon, sweetener, and the boiling coffee. Stir until thick, add milk, let cook 15 minutes, stirring with rotary beater. Cool and chill. Serve ice cold in tall glasses with whipped cream (optional) on top.

NUMBER OF SERVINGS: 4
TOTAL CARBO-CALORIES: 66
CARBO-CALORIES PER SERVING: 16½

EGGNOG

1 egg, separated
Artificial sweetener equivalent to 1 tablespoon sugar
½ teaspoon vanilla
1 cup hot milk
Nutmeg gratings

Beat egg yolk with sweetener until very light, add vanilla,
then add egg white, beaten stiff. Fill up the glass with the
hot milk. Put grated nutmeg on top. Serve hot or cold.

NUMBER OF SERVINGS: 1
TOTAL CARBO-CALORIES: 19
CARBO-CALORIES PER SERVING: 19

LEMONADE

Artificial sweetener equivalent to 2 tablespoons sugar
Juice ½ lemon
1 cup water

Mix and stir ingredients. Serve hot or cold.

NUMBER OF SERVINGS: 1
TOTAL CARBO-CALORIES: 3
CARBO-CALORIES PER SERVING: 3

HOT SPICED LEMONADE

Artificial sweetener equivalent to ½ cup sugar
½ teaspoon whole cloves
2-inch cinnamon bark
½ teaspoon allspice
Juice 4 lemons
1 lemon, sliced

Let 1 quart water, sweetener, and spices gradually come to a boil, simmer for 5 minutes and strain. When ready to use, add the lemon juice. Serve hot in punch glasses with a slice of lemon in each glass. Also good served ice cold.

NUMBER OF SERVINGS: 4
TOTAL CARBO-CALORIES: 12
CARBO-CALORIES PER SERVING: 3

HOT MALTED MILK WITH EGG

2 tablespoons malted milk
1 egg
⅔ cup hot milk
Few drops vanilla

Mix malted milk in cup to smooth paste with a little boiling water. Beat egg until light, add to malted milk, add hot milk and flavoring, stir until smooth, and serve.

NUMBER OF SERVINGS: 2
TOTAL CARBO-CALORIES: 26
CARBO-CALORIES PER SERVING: 13

MULLED WINE

1 quart claret
Artificial sweetener equivalent to 2 cups sugar
½ teaspoon whole cloves
1-inch cinnamon bark
1 lemon, sliced

Mix all ingredients and 1 cup water. Boil steadily for 15 minutes and strain. Serve hot.

NUMBER OF SERVINGS: 4
TOTAL CARBO-CALORIES: 88
CARBO-CALORIES PER SERVING: 22

PRUNE JUICE DRINK

½ cup prune juice
1 teaspoon lemon juice
Artificial sweetener to taste
¾ cup milk

Mix prune juice with lemon juice and sweetener. Add milk
gradually. Shake well.

NUMBER OF SERVINGS: 3
TOTAL CARBO-CALORIES: 27
CARBO-CALORIES PER SERVING: 9

EXOTIC DISHES FROM AROUND THE WORLD

ANTICUCHOS
(Roasted Bull's Heart)—Peru

1 beef heart (4 pounds)
1 cup vinegar
1 clove garlic, crushed
1 bay leaf
1 tablespoon parsley
Celery leaves
1 medium-sized onion, sliced
1 red pepper pod, crushed
1 teaspoon salt

Quarter the heart and let marinate overnight in a mixture of the ingredients listed. Then wipe dry, rub with garlic, sprinkle lightly with salt and pepper. It is usually spitted and broiled over an open fire. If desired, the heart may be cut into small pieces, skewered, and broiled in the oven till done.

NUMBER OF SERVINGS: 12
TOTAL CARBO-CALORIES: 183
CARBO-CALORIES PER SERVING: 15¼

BACALHAU À PORTUGUESE
(Portuguese Codfish)—Portugal

1 *pound onions, sliced ½ inch thick*
1 *pound potatoes, sliced ½ inch thick*
1 *pound dried codfish (soaked for 12 hours in 3 changes of water)*
1 *pound tomatoes, sliced ½ inch thick*
4 *medium-sized green peppers, sliced*
1 *tablespoon salt*
¼ *teaspoon pepper*
12 *sprigs parsley*
1 *cup olive oil*

Place a layer of onions at the bottom of a large pot. Cover with a layer of potatoes. Upon this place a layer of codfish, cut into squares about the size of the potatoes. Cover with a layer of tomatoes and a layer of peppers. Sprinkle with salt and pepper. Repeat layers until all vegetables and fish are used. Place parsley on top. Pour olive oil over contents of pot. Cover tightly and place over a low flame. Do not stir but shake pot occasionally. After ½ hour, test with a fork to see if ingredients are tender. Reduce flame and simmer for 15 minutes more or until done.

NUMBER OF SERVINGS: 10
TOTAL CARBO-CALORIES: 230
CARBO-CALORIES PER SERVING: 23

BARQUETTES D'HUÎTRES À LA NORMANDE
(Oyster Barquettes)—France

2½ *cups sifted flour*
½ *teaspoon salt*
¾ *cup butter*
⅓ *cup cold water*

Mix flour and salt. Cut in butter with two knives and mix evenly. Add ⅓ cup cold water gradually. Place dough in a dish and let stand in refrigerator for 1 hour. Roll out ⅛ inch thick and cut 12 pieces, then form into shell shapes. Bake shells at 450° F. for about 15 minutes.

12 large mushrooms
12 large shrimp
½ cup minced clams
24 fresh oysters
½ cup white wine
3 tablespoons butter
Salt
Dash cayenne
1 tablespoon lemon juice
1 egg yolk
2 tablespoons parsley for garnish

Cook mushrooms and shrimp separately and slice them. Cook clams and mince them. Mix mushrooms, shrimp, and clams. Poach oysters in their own liquor for 2 minutes. Remove from liquid and boil down liquid to ½ cup. Add white wine. Gradually add butter, whipping constantly. Add salt, cayenne, and lemon juice. Remove from flame and add egg yolk. Partially fill the pastry shells with the seafood mixture and place 2 oysters in each shell. Pour a little sauce over the barquettes and set briefly in a very hot oven, 450° F. Garnish with fresh parsley and arrange on a dish covered with a folded napkin.

NUMBER OF SERVINGS: 12
TOTAL CARBO-CALORIES: 642
CARBO-CALORIES PER SERVING: 53½

BORJÚPÖRKÖLT
(Braised Veal)—Hungary

2 large onions, chopped
4 tablespoons beef fat
4 pounds shoulder of veal, cubed
1 teaspoon salt
4 tablespoons paprika
1 cup sour cream

Brown onions in fat. Add veal, salt, and paprika, and let the meat brown in this mixture. Cover and let simmer for about an hour or until the meat is tender. Some water may be added when necessary. Stir the sour cream in 5 minutes before serving.

NUMBER OF SERVINGS: 12
TOTAL CARBO-CALORIES: 222
CARBO-CALORIES PER SERVING: 18½

BRUSSELS LOF
(Buttered Endives)—Holland

12 endives
½ cup creamed butter
Nutmeg

Cook endives in boiling salted water until tender. Take care that they remain whole. Drain endives and place on a hot platter. Cover with creamed butter. Sprinkle with nutmeg, or serve nutmeg separately.

NUMBER OF SERVINGS: 12
TOTAL CARBO-CALORIES: 72
CARBO-CALORIES PER SERVING: 6

CARIUCHO
(Steak with Sauce)—Ecuador

3 large onions
4 tablespoons oil
3 large tomatoes, chopped
2 green peppers, sliced
3 cups milk
4 tablespoons peanut butter
3 pounds steak
Salt, pepper, and paprika

Slice onions and fry in oil until slightly done. Add tomatoes and peppers and continue cooking over a low flame for 10 minutes. Add milk and peanut butter. Cover and simmer for ½ hour. Broil steak and season. Place on a platter and cover with the sauce. Place in a hot oven for a few minutes before serving.

NUMBER OF SERVINGS: 12
TOTAL CARBO-CALORIES: 360
CARBO-CALORIES PER SERVING: 30

CERKES TAVUGU
(Circassian Chicken)—Turkey

1 chicken (5 pounds)
1 large onion, quartered
1 medium-sized carrot
1 bunch parsley
1 teaspoon salt
Pepper
2 cups shelled walnuts
1 tablespoon paprika
3 slices white bread

Place chicken in pot and cover with water. Add onion, carrot, parsley, salt and pepper. Bring to a boil and skim off foam on top. Cover and cook until chicken is tender. Remove from pot and allow to cool. Save stock. When cool, remove skin and bones, and cut chicken into small pieces. Put walnuts through grinder twice. Save red walnut oil for garnish. Add paprika. Soak bread in chicken stock. Squeeze dry and add to walnuts and paprika. Mix well. Run bread-paprika-walnut mixture through grinder three times. Add 1 cup of chicken stock. Work into paste. Divide paste in half. Use one half to coat pieces of chicken. Arrange chicken in bowl and spread other half of paste over it. Sprinkle with additional paprika and drops of walnut oil. Serve cold.

NUMBER OF SERVINGS: 12
TOTAL CARBO-CALORIES: 270
CARBO-CALORIES PER SERVING: 22½

CHOCLOTANDAS
(Steamed Corn)—Ecuador

6 young ears of corn with husks
3 eggs, beaten
¼ cup lard
¼ cup butter
Artificial sweetener equivalent to 1½ tablespoons sugar
¼ pound cream cheese
Salt

Remove husks from corn carefully and set aside. Scrape the uncooked kernels from the cobs and grind them. Force them through a strainer. Add the eggs. Soften lard and butter and add this to the corn and eggs. Add sweetener, cream cheese, and salt. Mix well. Divide into 6 portions. Wrap each portion in a corn husk. Place wrapped portions on a rack and steam for 1 hour.

NUMBER OF SERVINGS: 6
TOTAL CARBO-CALORIES: 198
CARBO-CALORIES PER SERVING: 33

DÁL
(Lentils)—India

2 cups lentils
3 medium onions
2 cloves garlic, minced
¼ pound butter
1½ teaspoons curry powder
1 teaspoon salt
Artificial sweetener equivalent to 1 teaspoon sugar
Pinch red pepper
½ teaspoon chili powder

Soak lentils in cold water overnight, or for 12 hours. Fry sliced onions and garlic in butter till brown. Add a little water, curry powder, lentils, and remaining dry ingredients.

Let simmer over a low flame for about 10 minutes, stirring frequently. Add 2 cups hot water to mixture. Cook until lentils are tender but not mushy.

NUMBER OF SERVINGS: 6
TOTAL CARBO-CALORIES: 186
CARBO-CALORIES PER SERVING: 31

EBI NO TERIAKI
(Broiled Lobster)—Japan

3 lobsters (1½ pounds each)
1 tablespoon salt
5 tablespoons soy sauce
1 tablespoon sherry
½ teaspoon red pepper

Boil lobsters for 20 minutes in salt water. Cool. Remove legs. Cut each lobster lengthwise, halfway through, and put in the sauce made by mixing soy and sherry. Broil at a distance of 4 inches from fire. Repeat application of sauce several times. When lobster is done, sprinkle with red pepper.

NUMBER OF SERVINGS: 3
TOTAL CARBO-CALORIES: 60
CARBO-CALORIES PER SERVING: 20

FASOULIA
(Steamed Green Beans)—Egypt

1½ pounds green beans
½ medium-sized carrot
1 medium-sized green pepper
1 medium-sized onion
1 medium-sized tomato
1½ tablespoons butter
1 clove garlic
½ teaspoon salt

Clean vegetables and cut beans, carrot, and green pepper into long thin silvers. Chop onion and tomato into fine pieces. Put vegetables, butter, and garlic into a well-covered pot and steam over low flame. Add salt. Cook until tender.

NUMBER OF SERVINGS: 12
TOTAL CARBO-CALORIES: 48
CARBO-CALORIES PER SERVING: 4

FONDS D'ARTICHAUTS GRATINÉS À LA REINE
(Stuffed Hearts of Artichoke)—France

12 artichoke hearts
¼ cup butter
¼ cup flour
2 cups light cream
1 tablespoon salt
¼ teaspoon pepper
2 cups boiled chicken, shredded
4 tablespoons grated Parmesan cheese
¼ pound melted butter

Cook artichoke hearts for about 15 minutes and drain. Blot them dry and continue cooking till tender, by steaming in butter. Prepare a cream sauce by melting the ¼ cup butter in a saucepan or double boiler. Remove from heat and stir in flour. Return to flame and add cream gradually, stirring constantly as the mixture thickens. Cook about 3 minutes more and add seasoning. Mix half the cream sauce with boiled chicken. When the artichokes are tender, stuff them with the chicken mixture. Arrange the hearts on a buttered pan and cover with balance of cream sauce. Sprinkle with Parmesan cheese and melted butter and bake in hot oven, 450° F., for a few minutes.

NUMBER OF SERVINGS: 12
TOTAL CARBO-CALORIES: 324
CARBO-CALORIES PER SERVING: 27

FRIKADELLER
(Veal Balls)—Sweden

1 pound veal, finely ground
½ cup bread crumbs
1 egg, separated
½ teaspoon salt
¼ teaspoon pepper
½ cup chopped parsley
½ pound mushrooms, minced
2 tablespoons butter
½ cup bouillon

Mix ground meat with crumbs, egg yolk, salt and pepper, parsley, and mushrooms. Beat egg white till stiff and fold into mixture. Form small balls. Cook on slow fire for ½ hour in butter and bouillon. If desired, fry balls in butter until brown on all sides.

NUMBER OF SERVINGS: 6
TOTAL CARBO-CALORIES: 90
CARBO-CALORIES PER SERVING: 15

GALINHA CÓRADA
(Pink Chicken)—Portugal

2 tablespoons salt
1 tablespoon paprika
¼ pound butter
1 chicken (5 pounds)
4 slices bacon
1 tumbler Madeira
Chopped parsley for garnish

Mix salt and paprika with butter and rub chicken with mixture inside and out. Place in a roasting pan, breast up. Cover breast with bacon slices. Roast in medium oven, 350° F., for about 1½ hours, until nicely browned. Cover pan and continue cooking for 15 minutes. Pour wine over chicken and cover pan again. Reduce heat to 325° F., and cook 15 minutes more. Place on a hot platter and garnish with parsley.

NUMBER OF SERVINGS: 10
TOTAL CARBO-CALORIES: 335
CARBO-CALORIES PER SERVING: 33½

GÄNSEBRATEN
(Roast Goose)—Germany

1 goose (8 pounds)
Salt
Marjoram
3 tablespoons fat

Clean and wash goose. Salt inside and out. Rub inside with marjoram. Let stand for 2 hours. Cover bottom of roasting pan with ½ cup of hot water and 2 tablespoons fat. Brush bird with 1 tablespoon fat, melted. Place goose in pan, breast down, and cover. Roast in oven at 375° F. for 1 hour. Turn over and roast for another 30 minutes. Remove lid. Baste frequently with pan gravy. Add a little hot water if necessary. Skim off fat from time to time. Allow 15 minutes for each pound of ready-to-cook weight. During the last 15 minutes, increase oven heat to 450° F. to make skin crisp. Goose should be well done.

NUMBER OF SERVINGS: 16
TOTAL CARBO-CALORIES: 676
CARBO-CALORIES PER SERVING: 42¼

GEBACKENE PILZE
(Baked Mushrooms)—Austria

½ pound dried mushrooms
1 cup milk
2 medium-sized onions, chopped
2 tablespoons butter
Salt and pepper to taste
1 tablespoon sifted flour
2 cups sour cream
1 tablespoon chopped parsley for garnish

Wash mushrooms carefully in cold water and soak overnight in milk. Drain and dice mushrooms. Brown onions lightly in butter. Add mushrooms and cook over medium flame for 30 minutes. Add salt and pepper. Transfer mushrooms and onions to a buttered dish. Blend sifted flour with sour cream. Pour over mushrooms and sprinkle with parsley. Cover and bake at moderate heat, 350° F., for about 30 minutes.

NUMBER OF SERVINGS:	8
TOTAL CARBO-CALORIES:	104
CARBO-CALORIES PER SERVING:	13

GEBACKENER KARPFEN
(Fried Carp)—Austria

3 pounds carp fillet
Salt
¼ cup flour
2 eggs, beaten
6 tablespoons bread crumbs
¼ pound shortening (not butter)
1 lemon, sliced

Wash fish and cut into serving slices. Sprinkle with salt and let stand for 1 hour. Put flour, eggs, and bread crumbs in three separate dishes. Roll each slice of fish in flour, dip into eggs, and coat with bread crumbs. Fry each slice on both sides in shortening until golden brown. Arrange slices on a hot platter and garnish with lemon.

NUMBER OF SERVINGS: 10
TOTAL CARBO-CALORIES: 270
CARBO-CALORIES PER SERVING: 27

GEHAKTE LEBER
(Chopped Liver)—Israel

½ cup finely diced onions
½ cup melted chicken fat
1 pound chicken livers
2 hard-cooked eggs
Salt and pepper
Artificial sweetener equivalent to ¼ teaspoon sugar
1 tablespoon chopped dill

Fry diced onions in 2 tablespoons of chicken fat until tender and golden, but not browned. Add rest of fat and livers, which have been cut into 1-inch pieces. Fry for about 5 minutes. Place contents of pan in a wooden bowl. Add sliced eggs and chop all ingredients together. Season with salt, pepper, and sweetener. Chop well until mixture has the consistency of a smooth paste. Add finely chopped dill.

NUMBER OF SERVINGS: 8
TOTAL CARBO-CALORIES: 68
CARBO-CALORIES PER SERVING: 8½

GRÜNE BOHNEN
(String Beans)—Switzerland

1 pound string beans
½ medium onion, sliced
1 clove garlic, chopped
2 strips lean bacon, cubed
1 tablespoon butter
Salt and pepper

Cook string beans until done. Fry onion, garlic, and bacon in butter till onion is golden brown. Add salt and pepper and stir into string beans.

NUMBER OF SERVINGS: 4
TOTAL CARBO-CALORIES: 36
CARBO-CALORIES PER SERVING: 9

GUACAMOLE
(Mashed Avocados)—Mexico

4 avocados
2 small tomatoes, chopped
1 onion, chopped
1 teaspoon salt

Mash avocados into a smooth paste. Add the remaining ingredients. Mix well. This is used as a dipping for tortillas and as a garnish for tacos and all kinds of meats. It may also be used as an appetizer paste on crackers or toasted bread.

NUMBER OF SERVINGS: 16
TOTAL CARBO-CALORIES: 120
CARBO-CALORIES PER SERVING: 7½

HO SEE KOW YOOK FAT CHOY
(Dried Oysters with Pork and Seaweed)—China

1 pound dried oysters
½ pound pork tenderloin
½ cup soy sauce
1 teaspoon salt
1 clove garlic, crushed
¼ cup rice wine
1 cup peanut oil
½ ounce fat choy (dried seaweed)
2 cups chicken broth
1 small piece chicken fat
½ tablespoon cornstarch

Soak oysters in cold water for 2 hours till soft. Bring water to a boil, then strain and carefully clean all sand from the oysters. Again bring oysters to a boil in a saucepan, lower flame, and let oysters simmer for 10 minutes. Strain and save sauce (about ¼ cup). Wash pork tenderloin and wipe dry. Soak the whole piece in soy sauce with salt, garlic, and wine for 5 to 10 minutes. Deep fry it in hot oil until brown. Remove from flame. Run cold water over it for 10 to 20 minutes. Slice into ¼-inch-thick slices about the size of the oysters, and alternate pork slices and oysters in a bowl.

Wash seaweed, cover with chicken broth, and boil for 4 minutes with chicken fat. Strain and place on top of pork and oysters.

With 2 tablespoons of water, make a paste of the cornstarch. Add it to the sauce saved from the oysters and bring to a boil. Pour boiling sauce on top of the seaweed and serve.

NUMBER OF SERVINGS: 4
TOTAL CARBO-CALORIES: 102
CARBO-CALORIES PER SERVING: 25½

JANSSON'S FRESTELSE
(Jansson's Temptation)—Sweden

5 medium potatoes, boiled
15 anchovies
2 small onions, sliced
3 tablespoons butter
½ cup bread crumbs
Juice from anchovies
Pepper
1½ cups cream

Peel and slice potatoes lengthwise into thin strips. Cut anchovies into small pieces. Sauté onions lightly in 1 tablespoon of butter. Butter and crumb a baking dish and arrange potatoes and anchovies in alternate layers. Sprinkle each layer with anchovy juice and a dash of pepper. Dot with butter.

Pour the cream over the top. Bake in oven at 375° F. for 25 minutes. Reduce heat to 300° F. and continue baking for another 45 minutes or until done. Serve hot from baking dish.

NUMBER OF SERVINGS: 5
TOTAL CARBO-CALORIES: 175
CARBO-CALORIES PER SERVING: 35

KAKAVIÁ
(Fish Soup)—Greece

1 *whiting (1 pound)*
2 *large tomatoes, sliced*
½ *cup olive oil*
1 *pound onions, sliced*
1 *teaspoon salt*
¾ *pound haddock, sliced*
¾ *pound sea bass, sliced*
½ *pound shrimp*
2 *medium potatoes, sliced*
Salt and pepper

Clean whiting, leaving skin, head, and tail on. Place in heavy pot, together with tomatoes, oil, onions, and 1 teaspoon salt. Cover with water, bring to a boil, and simmer over low flame for 1 hour. Strain liquid and force whiting, tomatoes, and onions through a coarse sieve. Return fish stock and sieved ingredients to pot. Add rest of fish, as well as shrimp. Add potatoes. Boil 15 to 20 minutes. Add salt and pepper to taste.

NUMBER OF SERVINGS: 9
TOTAL CARBO-CALORIES: 171
CARBO-CALORIES PER SERVING: 19

KEPTA VERŠIENA
(Marinated Veal Roast)—Lithuania

1 veal roast (4 pounds)
1 medium-sized carrot
1 medium-sized onion
3 tablespoons dry mustard
Salt
6 strips bacon
1 tablespoon butter
3 tablespoons sour cream
½ tablespoon flour
Pan drippings from meat

Wash meat and dry it. Grate carrot and onion. Mix well with mustard. Rub mixture into the meat until it is absorbed. Place meat in a bowl, covered with a heavy plate so that meat is pressed down. Keep in refrigerator for 4 to 5 days. Before roasting, salt the meat. Place bacon on meat, and roast. Add butter and a few tablespoons of hot water to pan and place in moderate oven, 350° F. Allow 20 to 30 minutes per pound of meat. Baste meat frequently with pan drippings. When tender remove meat from oven and prepare gravy by mixing well the sour cream, flour, and pan drippings from the meat. Pour over meat and place back in oven to get a golden brown coloring.

NUMBER OF SERVINGS: 12
TOTAL CARBO-CALORIES: 198
CARBO-CALORIES PER SERVING: 16½

KIMCHI
(Pickled Vegetables)—Korea

2 pounds garden lettuce or cabbage
2 large white radishes
½ cup salt
1 whole small garlic, finely chopped
3 tablespoons finely chopped green onion
3 tablespoons finely chopped red peppers
1 tablespoon salt

Wash lettuce and peel radishes. Cut lettuce crosswise in strips of about 1½ inches. Slice radishes thin. Mix with lettuce. Sprinkle with ½ cup of salt and cover with 4 cups of water. Let stand for 10 hours. Wash and drain mixture thoroughly. Add garlic, onion, and peppers. Mix. Place in a pot with a tight-fitting lid. Add 1 tablespoon of salt and let stand in a warm place 2 to 3 days. After this it is ready to eat. Keep in refrigerator.

NUMBER OF SERVINGS: 8
TOTAL CARBO-CALORIES: 58
CARBO-CALORIES PER SERVING: 7¼

KOPŪSTAI SU GRYBAIS
(Sauerkraut with Mushrooms)—Lithuania

12 large dried mushrooms
6 strips bacon
1 onion, chopped
2 cups sauerkraut
1 tart apple, chopped
Salt

Soak mushrooms for 2 hours, then wipe dry and slice. Cut bacon into small pieces and brown onion with bacon lightly. Place sauerkraut and some of its own juice in a baking dish. Add bacon, onion, and apple. Add mushrooms and enough water to cover ingredients. Sprinkle with salt and cover baking dish. Place in a moderate oven for 3 hours.

NUMBER OF SERVINGS: 4
TOTAL CARBO-CALORIES: 60
CARBO-CALORIES PER SERVING: 15

LAVRAKI
(Baked Fillet of Fish)—Greece

5 pounds of any sea-fish fillet
Salt and pepper to taste
4 large onions, chopped
½ pound butter
½ cup cream
Juice 1 lemon

Wash the fillets and place in a buttered ovenproof dish. Sprinkle with salt and pepper. Brown the onions in butter in another pan. Pour 1 cup water, butter, and onions on the fish and let simmer till liquid is absorbed. Add cream and allow to come to a boil. Remove from flame and sprinkle fish with salt and lemon juice. Bake in a medium oven 30 to 40 minutes.

NUMBER OF SERVINGS: 15
TOTAL CARBO-CALORIES: 300
CARBO-CALORIES PER SERVING: 20

LEBAN ZABADDY SALADA
(Yoghurt Salad)—Egypt

2 medium-sized cucumbers, sliced
2 scallions, sliced
3 red radishes, sliced thin
1 tablespoon olive oil
1 tablespoon vinegar
1 clove garlic, crushed
Salt and pepper
2 cups yoghurt
1 teaspoon minced mint

Wash and dice vegetables. Mix oil, vinegar, and garlic. Add
salt and pepper. Add to yoghurt and mix. Add mint. Stir in
vegetables.

NUMBER OF SERVINGS: 4
TOTAL CARBO-CALORIES: 58
CARBO-CALORIES PER SERVING: 14½

LEBERKNÖDELSUPPE
(Bouillon with Liver Dumplings)—Germany

2 slices white bread, crust removed
½ pound beef liver
¼ medium onion
2 eggs, separated
⅛ pound butter
1 teaspoon minced parsley
1 teaspoon salt
½ teaspoon pepper
6 cups bouillon

Soak bread in water. Squeeze dry. Run bread, liver, and
onion through a very fine grinder. Add beaten egg yolks, butter, parsley, salt, and pepper. Mix well. Beat egg whites until
stiff, and fold into mixture. Make round dumplings and boil
in bouillon for about 10 minutes. Serve with bouillon.

NUMBER OF SERVINGS: 6
TOTAL CARBO-CALORIES: 105
CARBO-CALORIES PER SERVING: 17½

MAYERN CYMES
(Honeyed Carrots)—Israel

1½ pounds carrots
½ cup honey
¼ cup chicken fat or margarine
½ teaspoon salt
1 teaspoon cinnamon
Juice 1 lemon

Clean and cut carrots into very small pieces. Place in a sauce-pan with just enough water to cover carrots, and boil for 10 minutes. Add honey, fat, and salt. Cover and simmer gently over a low flame for at least 1 hour, stirring occasionally. When done, add cinnamon and lemon juice. Mix well. It should have a thick, creamy consistency. Serve with meat.

NUMBER OF SERVINGS:	12
TOTAL CARBO-CALORIES:	180
CARBO-CALORIES PER SERVING:	15

MURGI CURRY
(Chicken Curry)—India

2 stewing chickens (about 4 pounds each)
1 teaspoon salt
⅛ teaspoon dry red pepper
2 cups yoghurt
4 onions, sliced small
4 cloves garlic, minced
1-inch green ginger, minced
1 cup butter or fat
2 teaspoons coriander powder
1 teaspoon turmeric powder
1 teaspoon ground cumin seeds
½ teaspoon chili powder
½ teaspoon powdered mustard
1 teaspoon cinnamon
1 teaspoon crushed cloves
2 tomatoes, chopped
1 bouillon cube
Juice 1 lime or lemon

Clean and cut chicken into small sections. Sprinkle with salt and red pepper. Cover with yoghurt and let stand for ½ hour. Brown onions, garlic, and ginger in butter. Add other spices and mix well. Remove chicken from yoghurt and brown lightly in the butter, onion, etc., mixture. Add yoghurt and tomatoes and continue cooking over a brisk fire. Stir constantly until meat is brown and dry. Dissolve bouillon cube in 3 cups of boiling water and pour over chicken. Let simmer gently on low fire until chicken is tender. Add more water if necessary. About 10 minutes before chicken is done, squeeze lime juice over it.

NOTE: This dish is rather spicy for American taste. If a milder dish is desired, reduce amount of spices by one half.

NUMBER OF SERVINGS: 12
TOTAL CARBO-CALORIES: 552
CARBO-CALORIES PER SERVING: 46

OSASHIMI
(Sliced Fillet of Raw Fish)—Japan

1 pound sea bream or sole fillet
8 tablespoons soy sauce
Artificial sweetener equivalent to 2 tablespoons sugar
2 tablespoons vinegar
6 tablespoons grated horseradish

Cut fish on a slant into very thin (½-inch) slices. Blend soy sauce with sweetener and vinegar. Place sliced fish on small individual plates. Fish is eaten with horseradish and the soy sauce mixture.

NUMBER OF SERVINGS: 6
TOTAL CARBO-CALORIES: 39
CARBO-CALORIES PER SERVING: 6½

PAELLA VALENCIANA
(Chicken and Fish with Rice)—Spain

1 dozen shrimp
1 dozen mussels
2 small frying chickens, each cut into 8 pieces
½ pound lean pork
2 large Spanish onions, chopped fine
⅓ cup olive oil
1 tomato, skinned and crushed
1 clove garlic, crushed
1½ cups rice
¼ pound eel
Handful fresh lima beans
Handful sweet peas
2 bottoms of artichokes cut in quarters
2 sweet red peppers
3 cups sea-food liquid
½ bay leaf
Salt and pepper
¼ teaspoon saffron

Shell and cook shrimp and mussels. Save 3 cups of liquid. Paella is cooked in a heavy iron pot with a round bottom, called *paellera*. Any heavy pot with a tight cover may be substituted. Brown chicken, pork, and onions in olive oil; add tomato and garlic. Mix well. Add rice and fry 2 to 3 minutes. Add sea food and eel, lima beans, peas, artichokes, and red peppers. Pour the 3 cups of sea-food liquid over mixture and bring to boil. Add bay leaf, salt, pepper, and saffron. Cook over a brisk fire for 5 minutes, mixing frequently. Lower flame, cover pot, and simmer gently for 15 to 18 minutes or until rice absorbs the liquid and is quite dry. If baked, let cook in oven, 375° F., for 45 minutes. Serve with additional red peppers on top.

NUMBER OF SERVINGS: 8
TOTAL CARBO-CALORIES: 300
CARBO-CALORIES PER SERVING: 37½

PAPA RELLENA
(Stuffed Potatoes)—Peru

6 medium-sized potatoes
1½ pounds ground beef
2 tablespoons butter
1 large onion, sliced
1 clove garlic, crushed
Salt and pepper
3 large hard-cooked eggs
2 large eggs, beaten
⅓ cup flour
1 cup lard

Boil potatoes and mash. Sauté meat in butter in a skillet with onion. Add garlic and seasoning. Chop the eggs and add to meat mixture. Divide the meat mixture into 6 portions and roll into balls. Divide potatoes into 6 portions and mold around meat balls. Carefully roll balls first in beaten egg, then in flour. Use just enough flour to hold the egg. Fry balls in lard over low heat until golden brown. Serve hot.

NUMBER OF SERVINGS: 6
TOTAL CARBO-CALORIES: 366
CARBO-CALORIES PER SERVING: 61

PATLICAN DOLMASI
(Stuffed Eggplant)—Turkey

6 small round eggplants
Salt
2 large onions, chopped
⅔ cup olive oil
2½ cups rice, washed and partially dried
2 medium tomatoes, peeled and chopped
3 teaspoons chopped pine nuts
3 tablespoons black currants
1 teaspoon chopped mint
Artificial sweetener equivalent to 2 teaspoons sugar
Salt and pepper

Cut off stem ends of eggplants and save. Peel eggplants lengthwise, leaving strips of peel between cuts, so that peeled and unpeeled strips alternate. Scoop out the insides, leaving a shell of about 1 inch thickness. Sprinkle with salt and let stand. Brown onions lightly over a low flame in 3 tablespoons of oil. Add remaining oil and rice. Cook gently for 10 minutes. Add 1 cup water, tomatoes, pine nuts, currants, mint, sweetener, and salt and pepper to taste. Continue cooking for 10 minutes. Wash salt off eggplants, fill with stuffing, and replace stem ends to cover. Cover eggplants halfway with water in a pan. Cover pan tightly and stew for 45 minutes, or until tender. Serve cold.

NUMBER OF SERVINGS: 12
TOTAL CARBO-CALORIES: 276
CARBO-CALORIES PER SERVING: 23

POMODORI RIPIENI
(Stuffed Tomatoes)—Italy

9 small tomatoes, not too ripe
Pinch salt
1 can light meat tuna (7 ounces), mashed
18 anchovies, chopped
18 capers, crushed
3 tablespoons mayonnaise
1 tablespoon chopped parsley
3 hard-cooked eggs

Wash tomatoes and dry. Cut in half. Scoop out seeds and sprinkle with salt. Chill in refrigerator for ½ hour. Blend tuna, anchovies, and capers with mayonnaise. Fill each tomato half with the mixture. Sprinkle with parsley and garnish with sliced eggs.

NUMBER OF SERVINGS: 18
TOTAL CARBO-CALORIES: 108
CARBO-CALORIES PER SERVING: 6

RISENGRØD
(Rice Porridge)—Denmark

¾ pound rice
2 quarts milk
¼ teaspoon salt
¼ pound sweet butter
1 cup malt beer (dark)
2 cups sweet fruit juice

Wash rice and scald with boiling water. Drain. Bring ½ cup of cold water to boil in a saucepan. Pour in the milk. Bring milk and water to a slow boil over a low flame. Gradually pour in the washed and scalded rice, stirring constantly until the porridge boils. Cover the saucepan and let simmer over a low flame for about 1 hour. Season with salt. Apportion rice into individual plates. Put a pat of cold butter on top of each serving. Add heated malt beer. Mix fruit juice with ½ cup of water and heat slightly. Pour over the rice.

NUMBER OF SERVINGS:	12
TOTAL CARBO-CALORIES:	264
CARBO-CALORIES PER SERVING:	22

RØDKAAL
(Red Cabbage)—Denmark

2 pounds red cabbage
½ cup butter
Salt and sugar
1 tablespoon vinegar
Juice 1 lemon
½ cup red wine
1 tablespoon red currant juice

Wash cabbage and let stand for 1 hour in cold salted water. Drain. Slice the cabbage in long thin strips. Melt (but not brown) butter in a pot. Add a pinch of salt and sugar. Mix. Add the cabbage and slowly simmer for a few minutes. Cover pot and cook for about 2 hours or until very tender. Before serving, add vinegar, lemon juice, wine, red currant juice, and salt and sugar to taste. Red cabbage is best when prepared the day before it is served.

NUMBER OF SERVINGS:	8
TOTAL CARBO-CALORIES:	156
CARBO-CALORIES PER SERVING:	19½

RUNDERLAPPEN
(Spiced Beef)—Holland

3 pounds round steak, cut into 9 steaks
Salt and pepper
½ cup bacon drippings
3 medium onions, sliced
3 tablespoons vinegar
½ tablespoon dry mustard
1 bay leaf
½ teaspoon cloves
5 peppercorns

Scrape meat and rub each steak with salt and pepper. Heat bacon drippings in skillet until it is very hot. Brown meat thoroughly on both sides. Shortly before meat is done, add onions, which should be fried lightly but not browned. Place meat in a covered baking dish. To fat and onions in skillet add 1 cup water, vinegar, mustard, bay leaf, cloves, and peppercorns. Bring to a boil and pour over meat. Cover meat and allow to simmer very gently 2 to 3 hours at 350° F. until very soft. Turn meat every ½ hour.

NUMBER OF SERVINGS:	9
TOTAL CARBO-CALORIES:	252
CARBO-CALORIES PER SERVING:	28

SALADA DE QUIABOS
(Okra Salad)—Brazil

2 pounds okra
2 tablespoons olive oil
1 tablespoon vinegar
1 teaspoon finely grated onion
Salt and pepper

Select young, uniformly shaped okra. Cut off ends. Cover with salted water and boil 15 to 20 minutes until tender. Drain. Cool. Mix oil, vinegar, onion, salt, and pepper. Pour over okra.

NUMBER OF SERVINGS:	8
TOTAL CARBO-CALORIES:	36
CARBO-CALORIES PER SERVING:	4½

SALÁTA SAVANJUTÉFELLEL
(Lettuce in Sour Cream)—Hungary

1 head lettuce
1 cup sour cream
1 tablespoon vinegar
Salt and pepper
Paprika

Remove outer leaves of lettuce and trim browned edges. Cut heart in four pieces. Cook lettuce in salt water for 15 minutes. Wash and drain again. Place in a deep dish and pour sour cream, vinegar, salt, and pepper over it. Mix well and serve. It may be lightly sprinkled with paprika.

NUMBER OF SERVINGS:	4
TOTAL CARBO-CALORIES:	34
CARBO-CALORIES PER SERVING:	8½

SCALOPPINE DI VITELLO
(Veal Cutlets)—Italy

1 tablespoon butter
1½ pounds thin veal cutlets (about 10)
Slice of ham (boiled or precooked) for each cutlet
Slices of mozzarella, muenster, or Swiss cheese (1 for each cutlet)
½ cup chicken or beef stock (or bouillon)
Juice ½ lemon
1 teaspoon minced parsley

Butter a small casserole. Place layer of veal cutlets on bottom. Cover with layer of ham and layer of cheese. Pour stock and lemon juice over this. Dot with remaining butter. Bake at 375° F. for 1 hour. Sprinkle with parsley and serve.

NUMBER OF SERVINGS: 5
TOTAL CARBO-CALORIES: 100
CARBO-CALORIES PER SERVING: 20

SJØØRRET MED SMELTET SMØR
(Trout with Melted Butter)—Norway

1 fresh trout (4 pounds)
½ cup vinegar
1½ teaspoons salt
1 lemon, sliced
3 tablespoons chopped parsley
¼ pound butter
1 tablespoon lemon juice

Clean fish, leaving head and tail. Rinse with cold water. Place fish in a dish. Warm vinegar and pour over fish. Cover and let stand for 1 hour. In a large pot, bring to a boil 2½ quarts of salted water. Place the whole fish in the water and see that it is well covered with water. Cook fish on a slow fire for about 20 minutes, until meat can be easily separated from bones but does not fall apart. Lift fish carefully out of water and place on a large, hot platter. Garnish with lemon slices and half of the chopped parsley. Melt, but do not brown butter. Add remaining parsley and lemon juice and serve hot in a separate dish with the fish.

NUMBER OF SERVINGS: 8
TOTAL CARBO-CALORIES: 210
CARBO-CALORIES PER SERVING: 26¼

SOPA DE COUVE-FLOR
(Cauliflower Soup)—Brazil

1 large cauliflower
Salt
3 eggs, separated
2 tablespoons wheat flour
1 tablespoon grated Parmesan cheese
6 cups clear soup stock

Wash cauliflower thoroughly. Place in enough boiling water to cover. Add salt and let simmer gently for ½ hour. Remove from heat and drain water. Beat egg yolks. Add sifted flour, cheese, and a pinch of salt. Cook mixture in double boiler until slightly thickened. Beat egg whites until stiff and fold into mixture. Continue cooking for 5 minutes. Remove from heat immediately. Place sections of cauliflower in individual soup plates. Cover with sauce and pour hot soup stock over it.

NUMBER OF SERVINGS: 6
TOTAL CARBO-CALORIES: 45
CARBO-CALORIES PER SERVING: 7½

SOPA DE ESPINACA CON CODITO
(Spinach Soup with Macaroni)—Mexico

½ pound spinach
¼ pound elbow macaroni
½ onion, minced
2 tablespoons vegetable oil
½ cup tomato sauce
6 cups beef broth or bouillon
Salt and pepper
4 tablespoons butter

Boil spinach and macaroni separately; rinse and drain. Brown onion in oil and add tomato sauce. Stir and let simmer for 2 minutes. Add broth. Salt and pepper to taste. Bring the mixture to a boil and add macaroni. Then add the spinach and simmer for 5 minutes. When ready to serve, add butter and let simmer again for about 5 minutes.

NUMBER OF SERVINGS: 6
TOTAL CARBO-CALORIES: 78
CARBO-CALORIES PER SERVING: 13

SOPA DE PESCADO
(Fish Soup)—Spain

½ dozen shrimp
1 large Spanish onion, chopped
¼ cup olive oil
1 tomato, quartered
2 peppercorns, crushed
1 clove garlic, minced
1 bay leaf
1 sprig parsley, minced
1 fish head
2 pounds halibut
1½ pounds whitefish
Salt
3 pieces toast cut in squares

Wash shrimp and cover with boiling salted water. Simmer 10 to 15 minutes or until shells turn pink. Shell, saving liquid. Brown onion in oil in a separate pan. Add tomato, peppercorns, garlic, bay leaf, and parsley. Cover with boiling water, add fish head, and cook over hot flame for several minutes. Lower flame and simmer for another 10 minutes. Add sliced halibut, whitefish, and cut-up shrimp. Add liquid in which shrimp has been boiled. Be careful to avoid sand which may have accumulated at the bottom of pot. Continue cooking for 20 minutes. Season to taste with salt. Strain fish broth. Remove fish head. Place a few squares of toast, shrimp, and slices of fish in individual soup dishes. Pour broth over them. Serve.

NUMBER OF SERVINGS: 6
TOTAL CARBO-CALORIES: 138
CARBO-CALORIES PER SERVING: 23

STEKT KYLLING
(Chicken in Sour Cream Gravy)—Norway

2 chickens, small fryers, cut for frying
Salt and pepper
¼ pound butter
3 cups milk
2 tablespoons chopped parsley
¼ cup sherry
1½ cups sour cream

Season chicken with salt and pepper. Fry in butter until golden brown. Place chicken and drippings in a casserole. Cover with milk. Cook very slowly for about 30 minutes until tender. Add parsley and sherry and cook 5 to 10 minutes more. Add sour cream and stir into gravy. Keep in oven for 5 more minutes. Serve.

NUMBER OF SERVINGS: 8
TOTAL CARBO-CALORIES: 230
CARBO-CALORIES PER SERVING: 28¾

TIEM SHUEN YU
(Sweet and Sour Fish)—China

1 fresh sea bass (2 pounds)
½ teaspoon salt
½ cup water chestnut flour
1 egg
4 tablespoons cornstarch
⅔ cup peanut oil
1½ cups vinegar
Artificial sweetener equivalent to ½ cup sugar
½ teaspoon salt
1 tablespoon soy sauce
½ ounce fresh lemon rind
1 slice canned pineapple

Clean fish thoroughly and slice along back to remove bones. Salt the inside and outside of the fish. Make a batter of chestnut flour, egg, and 2 tablespoons cornstarch. Dip fish into batter. Deep fry in hot oil for 4 minutes until brown but not burned. Remove and place in a flat pan. With a little water, make a paste of the remaining cornstarch. Add vinegar, sweetener, ½ teaspoon salt, soy sauce, lemon rind, ½ cup water, and pineapple. Bring mixture to a boil in a saucepan. Pour over fish and allow to simmer for 15 minutes over low flame. Serve hot.

NUMBER OF SERVINGS: 6
TOTAL CARBO-CALORIES: 255
CARBO-CALORIES PER SERVING: 42½

TOLAN KOOK
(Soup with Beef and Sweet Potatoes)—Korea

2 pounds beef
2 pounds thick seaweed
Salt and pepper
2 pounds small sweet potatoes
Soy sauce

Cook beef and seaweed with salt and pepper in a pot of water for 4 hours. Add whole sweet potatoes and cook until done. Add soy sauce and salt to taste. Serve in a large plate with sliced beef, potatoes, and seaweed.

NUMBER OF SERVINGS:	12
TOTAL CARBO-CALORIES:	348
CARBO-CALORIES PER SERVING:	29

ZÜRCHER LEBERSPIESSLI
(Grilled Calf's Liver with Bacon on Skewers)—Switzerland

2 pounds calf's liver
Pepper
20 sage leaves, fresh or dried (crushed sage may be used)
6 thin slices bacon
¼ cup butter
Salt
3 tablespoons hot bouillon

Remove the skin from the liver. Cut into thin slices and sprinkle lightly with pepper. Cut into 1½-inch strips. Sprinkle each strip with sage, or place ½ leaf on each strip. Divide the bacon lengthwise and wrap each piece of liver with a strip of bacon and place on skewers, 5 or 6 pieces to each skewer. Melt butter in a frying pan, but do not brown. Arrange skewers in the hot butter and cover. Fry over a medium flame about 10 to 12 minutes, or until liver is done. Add salt, and pour bouillon over liver. Remove liver from skewers after the bouillon has soaked in for 2 to 3 minutes, and place on hot platters.

NUMBER OF SERVINGS:	6
TOTAL CARBO-CALORIES:	90
CARBO-CALORIES PER SERVING:	15

Index